Rape Plots

Studies in Biblical Literature

Hemchand Gossai
General Editor

Vol. 13

PETER LANG
New York • Washington, D.C./Baltimore • Boston • Bern
Frankfurt am Main • Berlin • Brussels • Vienna • Canterbury

Susanne Scholz

Rape Plots

A Feminist Cultural Study
of Genesis 34

PETER LANG
New York • Washington, D.C./Baltimore • Boston • Bern
Frankfurt am Main • Berlin • Brussels • Vienna • Canterbury

Library of Congress Cataloging-in-Publication Data

Scholz, Susanne.
Rape plots: a feminist cultural study of Genesis 34 / Susanne Scholz.
p. cm. — (Studies in biblical literature; vol. 13)
Includes bibliographical references and index.
1. Rape in the Bible. 2. Bible. O.T. Genesis XXXIV—Feminist criticism. 3. Bible.
O.T. Genesis XXXIV—Criticism, interpretation, etc.—History. 4. Rape—
Religious aspects—Christianity—History. 5. Medical jurisprudence—
Germany—History—19th century. I. Title. II. Series.
BS1199.R27S36   220.8'3641532—dc21   98-40740
ISBN 0-8204-4154-6 (hardcover)
ISBN 0-8204-6107-5 (paperback)
ISSN 1089-0645

Die Deutsche Bibliothek-CIP-Einheitsaufnahme

Scholz, Susanne:
Rape plots: a feminist cultural study of Genesis 34 / Susanne Scholz.
–New York; Washington, D.C./Baltimore; Boston; Bern;
Frankfurt am Main; Berlin; Brussles; Vienna; Canterbury: Lang.
(Studies in biblical literature; Vol. 13)
ISBN 0-8204-4154-6 (hardcover)
ISBN 0-8204-6107-5 (paperback)

The paper in this book meets the guidelines for permanence and durability
of the Committee on Production Guidelines for Book Longevity
of the Council of Library Resources.

Printed in the United States of America

I do not weep at the world—I am too busy
sharpening my oyster knife.

Zora Neale-Hurston

Table of Contents

Editor's Preface

More than ever the horizons in biblical literature are being expanded beyond that which is immediately imagined; important new methodological, theological, and hermeneutical directions are being explored, often resulting in significant contributions to the world of biblical scholarship. It is an exciting time for the academy as engangement in biblical studies continues to be heightened.

This series seeks to make available to scholars and institutions, scholarship of a high order, which will make a significant contribution to the ongoing biblical discourse. This series includes established and innovative directions, covering general and particular areas in biblical study. For every volume considered for this series, we explore the question as to whether the study will push the horizons of biblical scholarship. The answer must be *yes* for inclusion.

In this volume, Susanne Scholz explores in an original new direction the study of Genesis 34 and the rape of Dinah. Her work demonstrates not only scholarship of the highest order, but an engagement with the text, and the sensibilities about sexual violence which sets this study apart. This volume will provide significant new insights in the interpretation of Genesis 34 and cast important new light on the manner in which this text in particular and the issue of rape in general must be reckoned with. Scholz's innovative analysis on rape and forensic medicine in nineteenth-century Germany is certain to take the discourse about rape into new and challenging avenues.

Scholz's study will take its place among other indispensable resources for anyone who seeks to pursue the study of Genesis 34, and the manner in which sexual violence is understood and responded to by the global community. The horizon has been expanded.

Hemchand Gossai
General Editor

Acknowledgments

This book is a slightly revised version of my Ph.D. thesis that I defended at Union Theological Seminary in the City of New York in May 1997. I was fortunate to quickly find a publisher, and I thank Hemchand Gossi, General Editor of Peter Lang Publishing, to accept my study in his series *Studies in Biblical Literature*. I am also grateful to Heidi Burns, Senior Editor, for her editorial support and comments.

Many people played a crucial role in the process of researching, writing, and finally publishing this work. First and foremost, I thank Phyllis Trible, Professor of Old Testament and Associate Dean at Wake Forest University in North Carolina and previously Baldwin Professor of Sacred Literature at Union Theological Seminary in the City of New York, for her continuous support, her relentless challenge toward clarity and simplicity in thought and writing, and her enduring encouragement during my years as her student at Union Theological Seminary. Her integrity and love for the Bible enabled me to pursue this work. I also thank the members of my dissertation committee for their valuable suggestions and support: Mary C. Boys and George M. Landes of Union Theological Seminary, Kathryn Gravdal and Atina Grossmann of Columbia University.

The study required research in several libraries. I benefited from the many libraries in New York City: the Burke Library of Union Theological Seminary, the libraries of Columbia University, especially the Health Sciences Library, the New York Academy of Medicine, the library of Jewish Theological Seminary, NY, and the New York Public Library. I also thank the staff of the National Library of Medicine, Bethesda, Maryland. During the publication stage the excellent services of the libraries at Fordham University, NY, and The College of Wooster, Ohio, enabled me to do the necessary final checks.

I extend my deep thanks to the World Council of Churches and Union Theological Seminary for awarding me with a scholarship and fellowships that financed the lion's share of an expensive but most valuable program. Thanks to the faculty of Union Theological Seminary. Special thanks to Beverly W. Harrison who made time when there was no time and encouraged interdisciplinary work through her own example. I thank Robert E. Seaver and Vincent L. Wimbush. Thanks also to Edward L. Greenstein, formerly at Jewish Theological Seminary, NY, and now at Tel Aviv University, Israel. I also thank my former professors in Germany, Rolf Rendtorff at the University of Heidelberg and Luise Schottroff at the Gesamthochschule Kassel who demonstrated through their own scholarship the gains of being involved in international scholarship. I am grateful to Erhard S. Gerstenberger at the University of Marburg who provided indispensable comments and suggestions for publishing the dissertation.

I benefited from presenting portions of my work at academic conferences which I gratefully acknowledge: the annual meetings of the Society of Biblical Literature (1995-1997), the annual meeting of the Feminist Friends of Ethics (1994), the Tenth Annual Klutznick Symposium in 1997, and the New Scholars in Gender Series at Bard College in 1997. I gratefully acknowledge Sheffield Academic Press for granting permission to reprint materials from my articles published in the following volumes; "Was It Really Rape in Genesis 34? Biblical Scholarship as a Reflection of Cultural Assumptions." In *Escaping Eden: New Feminist Perspectives on the Bible,* ed. Harold C. Washington, Susan Lochrie Graham and Pamela Thimmes, 182–198. Sheffield: Sheffield Academic Press, 1998; "Through Whose Eyes? A 'Right' Reading of Genesis 34." In *Genesis: A Feminist Companion to the Bible (Second Series),* ed. Athalya Brenner, 150–171. Sheffield: Sheffield Academic Press, 1998.

I thank three dear German friends, all Protestant ministers, who sent me material that I could not find in the United States: Ursula Bauer, Diemut Cramer, and Kathinka Kaden. Thanks to Yeong-Mee Lee for many conversations about life and work at Union. Many thanks also to Chris Herlinger who offered important editorial comments. During our cultural explorations in New York we noticed the pervasiveness of rape, even when nobody else did. I thank my family of origin for their encouraging letters, telephone calls, and visits since I crossed the ocean: Witha, Christine, Anni, Erika, Ekkehard and Gabi. Finally, I am profoundly grateful to Lorraine Keating. Talking to her in the car one rainy evening at a red light on Broadway, I conceived the idea for this study. Her persistent interest invigorated my own. Our conversations and mutual amazements about "rape plots" lightened and enlightened the project with laughter, insights, and a sense of sanity. Maybe this is the only way to immerse oneself in a somber topic like the one of the following pages.

October 31, 1998

Chapter 1

Introduction:
Rape, Culture, and Genesis 34

The Pervasiveness of Rape Today

Rape is an omnipresent threat for women in today's world. Friends
and family members rape women. They are raped in schools and sometimes even on travel seminars. Soldiers rape women indiscriminately
all over the world. Women don't feel safe anywhere—in parks or in
streets. Many movies treat the subject obliquely, but others such as
What's Love Got to Do With It? or *The Accused* portray rape quite
explicitly. And the media are filled with rape stories. A random list of
topical stories in *The New York Times* proves the case:

In the streets and in the family: "Police Officer Is Charged in Rape
of Bronx Girl, 17" (Aug. 9, 1996), "Six Attacks Reported over Week-
end" (Aug. 12, 1996), "Accuser Faces Rape Suspect, 10 Years Later"
(Oct. 16, 1996), "The Ritual Slaves of Ghana: Young and Female"
(Jan. 20, 1997), "A Woman's Shooting of Attacker Rivets Mexico"
(Feb. 5, 1997), ""Man Charged with Raping Date He Met from E-
Mail" (Feb. 24, 1997), "Sex-Slayings Alarm France on the Peril of
Repeat Offenders" (Feb. 25, 1997), Mother and Daughter Are Raped
in Woods" (June 16, 1997), "Murder Suspect Says He Felt 'Invincible'
after Park Rape" (Dec. 16, 1997), "Rape Suspect Pleads No Contest
in Nebraska" (Feb. 18, 1998), "Queens Man Is Charged In 2d Rape of
Daughters" (Feb. 26, 1998), "Women Raped at Gunpoint in Flushing
Meadows Park" (April 14, 1998), "Group Forced Illegal Aliens Into
Prostitution, U.S. Says" (April 24, 1998).

In the schools: "Girl, 15, Reports Another Student Raped Her"
(Sept. 17, 1996), "Four Teen-Agers Charged in Rape of Girl in a
Classroom in Queens" (May 21, 1997), "Withering Report Criticizes

Officials Over a Rape in School" (Sept. 17, 1997), "5 Maryland College Students Are Raped on Guatemala Trip" (Jan. 19, 1998).

In the military and in wars: "In Okinawa, U.S. Bases Remain a Big
Issue" (March 9, 1996), "Japan Pays Some Women from War Broth-
els, but Many Refuse" (Aug. 15, 1996), "Rape Trial of Male Cadet
under Way at West Point" (Jan. 22, 1997), "A War-Crime Trial, But of
Muslims, Not Serbs" (April 3, 1997), and finally "Rape Cases Shake
up the Army in Canada" (July 16, 1998). An excerpt of a sad litany.

But why is rape such a continuous threat to women of all ages,
classes, races, and ethnicities? Why do so many men rape so many
women as well as children and even other men?[1] For a quarter of a
century, feminists have attempted to explain this phenomenon. Susan
Brownmiller began the search for answers and solutions.[2] Since the
1970s publications on rape have increased enormously; rows of books
fill the stacks of libraries. In recent years researchers have become
interested in studying the cultural roots of rape. They have begun
investigating the connection between cultural expressions, such as art
and literature, and the occurrence of rape.[3] In the field of religion,
feminist scholars have researched the link between religion and rape.
For example, the contributions in *Violence Against Women and
Children: A Christian Theological Sourcebook* describe the enormous consequences of violence in the lives of women of faith.[4]

This study participates in the effort to explore the roots of rape in
Western-Christian history and culture, here in the discipline of biblical
scholarship. The fundamental question for the following chapters is:
How has biblical scholarship contributed to the contemporary prevalence of rape? The task is enormous and boundaries have to be set. I

---

[1] For an increasing awareness of men raping men see, e.g., "Prisoner's Cry of
Rape Is Heard" (New York Times Oct. 9, 1996), B1.

[2] Susan Brownmiller, *Against Our Will: Men, Women and Rape* (New York:
Bantam, 1975).

[3] Lynn A. Higgins and Brenda R. Silver, eds., *Rape and Representations* (New
York: Columbia University Press, 1991); Patricia Searles and Ronald J. Berger, eds.,
Rape and Society: Readings on the Problem of Sexual Assault (Boulder, CO:
Westview, 1995).

[4] Carol J. Adams and Marie Fortune, eds., *Violence against Women and Children: A Christian Theological Sourcebook* (New York: Continuum, 1995). See
also Elisabeth Schüssler Fiorenza and Mary Shawn Copeland, eds., *Violence Against
Women* (London: SCM Press, 1994); Marie M. Fortune, *Love Does Not Harm:
Sexual Ethics For the Rest of Us* (New York: Continuum, 1995).

chose a limited and particular area for the examination of biblical interpretations. My work is, therefore, a case study. Grounded in feminist theories on rape, this book examines Genesis 34 and its history of interpretation to demonstrate how readers of one particular biblical story have participated in a cultural discourse that apologized, evaded, and minimized the harm of rape. Several considerations led to my choice of Genesis 34. The narrative is a short text, contained in one chapter. The brevity lends itself to concise interpretations. Biblical scholarship, feminist or otherwise,[5] has not studied this chapter as extensively as others. Often considering Genesis 34 as an independent later source within the Jacob cycle, scholars neglected the story.[6] Yet Genesis 34 presents a particularly provocative story line because the consequences of the rape are meticulously described. Without this description scholars might not have disclosed their ideas about rape so clearly. For these reasons Genesis 34 constitutes an excellent way to examine how rape has been interpreted through biblical scholarship.

More broadly, it offers an excellent opportunity to illustrate the relationship between the Bible, biblical scholarship, and Western culture. In recent years several biblical scholars have emphasized the importance of connecting biblical studies and culture. For example, J. Cheryl Exum has stated that "perhaps no other document has been so instrumental as the Bible in shaping Western culture and influencing ideas about the place of women and about the relationship of the sexes."[7] Vincent L. Wimbush maintains that the Bible has "profoundly

---

[5] Note that the chapter is not interpreted in Phyllis Trible, *Texts of Terror* (Philadelphia: Fortress, 1984); Letty M. Russell, ed., *Feminist Interpretation of the Bible* (Philadelphia: Westminster Press, 1985); Katheryn Pfisterer Darr, *Far More Precious Than Jewels: Perspectives on Biblical Women* (Louisville, KY: Westminster/Knox Press, 1991); J. Cheryl Exum, *Fragmented Women: Feminist (Sub)Versions of Biblical Narratives* (Valley Forge, PA: Trinity Press International, 1993). For an analysis of interpretations of Genesis 34 by early Christian and medieval exegetes, see Lucille C. Thibodeau, "The Relation of Peter Abelard's 'Planctus Dinae' to Biblical Sources and Exegetic Tradition: A Historical and Textual Study" (Ph. D. diss., Harvard University, 1990).

[6] Michael Fishbane, "Composition and Structure in the Jacob Cycle (Gen. 25:19-35:22)," *Journal of Jewish Studies* 26 (1975): 15-38. See also the analysis of interpretations in chapter 5 in the section entitled "Focus on the Men: Jacob" and the beginning of chapter 6.

[7] J. Cheryl Exum, "Feminist Criticism: Whose Interests Are Being Served?," in *Judges and Method: New Approaches in Biblical Studies*, ed. Gale A. Yee (Minneapolis: Fortress, 1995), 66.

affected the imagination of western culture."[8] A group of scholars calling themselves "The Bible and Culture Collective" has stated that "the
Bible has exerted more cultural influence on the West than any other
single document."[9] The current interest in correlating biblical studies
and culture provides a setting for exploring possible connections between interpretations of Genesis 34 and the "rape culture" of Western societies.[10]

Rape Culture and the Bible

Feminists coined the phrase *rape culture* to capture the extent of
sexual violence against women in the industrialized world. They have
argued that sexual violence permeates every aspect of life, including
"TV programs and ads, newspapers, novels, poetry, song, opera, rock,
and rap, every billboard, every shop window, every museum wall."[11]
All these aspects reflect societal mechanisms that accept, promote,
and produce rape. The term "rape culture" expresses that not only
"sick individuals" commit rape but society as a whole encourages it.

Rape can be defined as the uninvited physical (genital or oral) attack on a woman, a child, or a man by one or several men. Rape lacks
the consent of the one attacked; it includes physical, verbal, or nonverbal intimidation, threat, and frequently violence. It is a behavior
that political, economic, and societal structures of violence and hierarchy perpetuate. In contemporary Western societies women are the
primary targets of rape by men in times of peace and war, but there is
also abundant evidence that children and men are raped, especially,
in the case of men who are imprisoned.

The Bible contains several descriptions of rape or threatened rape.
The rape threat of Sarah (Genesis 20; 26), the rape of Dinah (Genesis
34), the rape of the concubine (Judges 19-21), the rape of Tamar (2
Samuel 13), possibly the forced intercourse of Hagar (Genesis 16;

---

[8] Vincent L. Wimbush, "Biblical-Historical Study as Liberation: Toward an Afro-
Christian Hermeneutic," *Journal of Religious Thought* 42, no. 2 (Fall-Winter 1985-
1986): 15.

[9] The Bible and Culture Collective, *The Postmodern Bible* (New Haven, CT: Yale
University Press, 1995), 1.

[10] For the term "rape culture" see Emilie Buchwald, Pamela R. Fletcher, and
Martha Roth, eds., *Transforming a Rape Culture* (Minneapolis: Milkweed, 1993).

[11] Buchwald, Fletcher, Roth, *Rape Culture*, 2.

21), the threatened rape of the young woman Abishag (1 Kings 1), and possibly God's rape threat to the prophet Jeremiah (Jeremiah 20:7). The rape threat of the cities Jerusalem and Samaria (Ezekiel 16; 23) are prominent examples of an extended understanding of the act. Presentation and treatment of rape in these texts differ. For example, the concubine is betrayed by her husband who delivered her into the hands of the rapists outside the house. Almost dead, she remains silent (Judges 19:28). The rape leads to further violence. Her husband cuts her into pieces to fulfill his plan which in the end leads to the killing of most of the tribe of Benjamin and the abduction and subsequent rape of many young women.

In another story a raped woman speaks. Tamar pleads with her brother Amnon, "No, my brother, do not force me; for such a thing is not done in Israel; do not do anything so vile!" (2 Samuel 13:12; NRSV). After the rape she has nowhere to go in the king's house. She does not agree to be sent away: "No, my brother; for this wrong in sending me away is greater than the other that you did to me!" (2 Samuel 13:16a). In despair, she puts ashes on her head, tears her robe, and cries aloud. Her brother Absalom later kills Amnon, his brother, for the rape. Stories vary in their presentation, reflection, and treatment of rape.

Genesis 34 represents yet another way. Dinah, the daughter of Leah and Jacob, is raped by Shechem, the prince of the land, when she goes to visit women in her neighborhood. Desiring her after the rape, Shechem abducts Dinah and asks his father, Hamor, to assist him with his plan to marry her. In the meantime Dinah's father, Jacob and her brothers hear about the rape. The brothers react strongly. When Shechem and Hamor negotiate the marriage, the brothers request that all the Canaanite males in the town be circumcised. While the male Shechemites lie in pain after the circumcision, Dinah's brothers attack the city and kill all the males, including Shechem and Hamor; they then abduct the women and children of the city. When Jacob hears about these actions, he condemns his sons. They ask in return if their sister should be treated like a whore. With that question the story ends.

Location in Biblical Scholarship

The present study wants to challenge biblical scholars to be ethically accountable for the content and consequences of their interpretations of Genesis 34. The emphasis of readers and their readings has gained prominence in the emerging field of biblical cultural studies. During the last decade this field has emerged, informed by cultural studies as practiced in numerous academic disciplines.[12] Cultural studies explore the interrelationship among various facets of political, economic, social institutions, beliefs, and behavior within human communities. The growing prominence of cultural studies in universities,[13] the expanding membership in the biblical guild to include people traditionally excluded, and increasing efforts to relate biblical studies to contemporary societal issues have encouraged the turn to cultural criticism.[14]

In this pursuit biblical scholars investigate the significance of the Bible as "cultural heritage."[15] They compare biblical interpretations from different historical and social perspectives.[16] They hypothesize about the usage of the Bible in Western political and economic movements of expansion.[17] They juxtapose biblical themes with other cultural sources, such as film, art, literature, and music,[18] and they en-

---

[12] For an introduction see Vincent B. Leitch, *Cultural Criticism, Literary Theory, Poststructuralism* (New York: Columbia University Press, 1992).

[13] See Michel Foucault, *The Archaeology of Knowledge and the Discourse on Language*, trans. A. M. Sheridan Smith (New York: Pantheon Books, 1972); Vincent B. Leitch, *American Literary Criticism from the Thirties to the Eighties* (New York: Columbia University Press, 1988), 81-114, 115-47, 400-5.

[14] See, for example, Letty M. Russell, ed., *Feminist Interpretation of the Bible* (Philadelphia: Westminster Press, 1985); R. S. Sugirtharajah, ed., *Voices from the Margin: Interpreting the Bible in the Third World* (Maryknoll, NY: Orbis, 1991); Cain Hope Felder, ed., *Stony the Road We Trod: African American Biblical Interpretation* (Minneapolis: Fortress, 1991); Kwok Pui-lan, *Discovering the Bible in the Non-Biblical World* (Maryknoll, NY: Orbis, 1995).

[15] Wim Beuken and Sean Freyne, eds., *The Bible as Cultural Heritage*, Concilium 1 (Maryknoll, NY: Orbis, 1995).

[16] Theophus H. Smith, *Conjuring Culture: Biblical Formations of Black America* (New York: Oxford University Press, 1994); Brian K. Blount, *Cultural Interpretation: Reorienting New Testament Criticism* (Minneapolis: Fortress, 1995); Stephen Breck Reid, *Listening In: A Multicultural Reading of the Psalms* (Nashville, TN: Abingdon Press, 1997).

[17] Michael Prior, *The Bible and Colonialism: A Moral Critique* (Sheffield: Sheffield Academic Press, 1997).

[18] Bernard Brandon Scott, *Hollywood Dreams and Biblical Stories* (Minneapolis: Fortress, 1994); J. Cheryl Exum, *Plotted, Shot, and Painted: Cultural Representations of Biblical Women* (Sheffield: Sheffield Academic Press, 1996); Alice Bach, *Women, Seduction, and Betrayal in Biblical Narrative* (New York: Cambridge University Press, 1997).

gage in a metadiscourse how various groups interpret the Bible.[19] Testifying to the emergence of cultural studies, the first volume of *The New Interpreter's Bible* includes several introductory articles in which scholars describe different strategies for reading the Bible from various social locations. Such locations include those of women, African-Americans, Hispanics, Native Americans, Jews, or Christians. In these varied discussions about the significance of gender, class, race, and ethnicity for biblical scholarship[20] the focus turns to the context of interpreters, teachers, students, and lay readers of the Bible.[21]

"Real" readers inextricably belong to social contexts. These locations shape the way they read texts and the interpretations that evolve.[22] Cultural critics understand that no one reads from the vantage point of neutrality or impartiality. They reject objective, value-free, and universally valid reconstructions of the biblical past and focus on the impact of interpretations on culture and that of culture on interpretations. Hence, cultural biblical criticism has emerged as "a joint critical study of texts and readers, perspectives and ideology."[23]

Biblical scholars have pursued cultural criticism in different ways. Bernard Brandon Scott juxtaposes mythical themes of selected contemporary movies to the New Testament.[24] Integrating sociolinguistic theory into his analysis, Brian K. Blount describes culturally diverse readings of various biblical texts applied by the peasants of Solentiname, American black slaves and churches, and biblical scholars like Rudolph

---

[19] Fernando F. Segovia and Mary Ann Tolbert, eds., *Reading from This Place*, vol. 1: *Social Location and Biblical Interpretation in the United States*, vol. 2: *Social Location and Biblical Interpretation in Global Perspective* (Minneapolis: Fortress, 1995); The Bible and Culture Collective, *The Postmodern Bible* (New Haven, CT: Yale University Press, 1995).

[20] *The New Interpreter's Bible: A Commentary in Twelve Volumes*, vol. 1 (Nashville, TN: Abingdon Press, 1994), 150-87.

[21] Fernando F. Segovia, "'And They Began to Speak in Other Tongues': Competing Modes of Discourse in Contemporary Biblical Criticism," in *Reading from This Place*, vol. 1: *Social Location and Biblical Interpretation in the United States*, ed. Fernando F. Segovia and Mary Ann Tolbert (Minneapolis: Fortress, 1995), 28.

[22] Ibid., 13. For a popular scientific study of the impact on the reader, see Gary Taylor, *Cultural Selection* (New York: Basic Books, 1996), 18: "We *select* an experience for recollection, after *evolving* its importance to *us*." See also John Gribbin, *Schrödinger's Kitten and the Search for Reality: Solving the Quantum Mysteries* (Boston: Little, Brown, 1995).

[23] Segovia, "'And They Began," 29.

[24] Scott, *Hollywood Dreams*.

Bultmann to show that "there can never be one final text interpreta-tion."[25] A collection of essays by J. Cheryl Exum represents yet an-other way of "doing" biblical cultural criticism. Exum analyzes how paintings, operas, or movies portrayed biblical women, such as Bathsheba, Delilah, and Michal.[26]

Different from these works, the present study on Genesis 34 stresses the need of a moral-ethical concern for biblical cultural studies.[27] Fo-cusing on a single topic and a single text, the study begins by describ-ing feminist scholarship on rape and so creates a basis for the analysis of biblical scholarship. Then the study depicts ideas on rape present in biblical interpretations from the nineteenth century. Theories on rape by nineteenth-century forensic medicine follow. Correlating ideas of the commentaries to forensic medical texts of nineteenth-century Germany ensures that the views of the commentators cannot simply be dismissed for their religious-theological origin. The comparison with scientific views demonstrates that the commentaries did not emerge from isolation. Rather, they were part of a broader cultural discourse.

The Significance of a Cultural Context

This book maintains that the explicit establishment of a cultural con-text sustains an interpretive perspective and exegesis of a biblical text. Consequently, a chapter on feminist scholarship on rape defines the perspective through which biblical and forensic scholarship are exam-ined. However, it is not likely that feminist scholars tried to influence biblical scholars. Similarly, contemporary biblical commentaries dem-onstrate that biblical scholars did not read feminist research. Indeed, most contemporary biblical interpretations or feminist scholarship do

---

[25] Blount, *Cultural Interpretation*, 184. Interpretations from different contexts can be found in Jean-Pierre Ruiz, "New Ways of Reading the Bible in the Cultural Setting of the Third World," in *The Bible as Cultural Heritage*, ed. Wim Beuken and Seán Freyne (Maryknoll, NY: Orbis, 1995), 73-84.

[26] Exum, *Plotted*.

[27] For the importance of this concern see, for example, Elisabeth Schüssler Fiorenza, "The Ethics of Interpretation: De-Centering Biblical Scholarship," *Jour-nal of Biblical Literature* 107, no. 1 (March 1988): 3-17; Stephen Fowl, "The Ethics of Interpretation or What's Left Over After the Elimination of Meaning," in *The Bible in Three Dimensions: Essays in Celebration of Forty Years of Biblical Studies in the University of Sheffield*, ed. David J. A. Clines, Stephen E. Fowl, Stanley E. Porter (Sheffield: Sheffield Academic Press, 1990), 379-98.

not reflect a direct influence. Nevertheless, the description of feminist scholarship grounds the critique of biblical scholarship in an academically informed and explicitly stated perspective.

The chapter on forensic medical textbooks exemplifies the general cultural discourse on rape for commentaries of nineteenth-century Germany. The choice of forensic medicine builds on the work of the philosopher Michel Foucault who demonstrated that the discourse on sexuality developed in the field of medicine during the nineteenth century.[28]

The choice of forensic medicine does not exclude other possibilities. In fact, other sources, such as legal documents, art, or literature might have been equally representative. Furthermore, the relationship posited between context and interpretations is not based upon the principle of cause and effect. The relationship does not assume direct links between biblical interpretations and the chosen setting. Specifically, the parallel between forensic medical textbooks and biblical commentaries of nineteenth-century Germany does not imply that biblical scholars actually read the textbooks. Likewise, it is doubtful that forensic authors tried to influence biblical scholars. Biblical interpretations or forensic textbooks indicate no evidence of such a direct influence; they do not tell us from where they derived their ideas. They illustrate that prejudices against raped women prevailed indeed beyond biblical scholarship.

Correlations between interpretations and context assume that the ideas about rape in biblical scholarship did not develop in isolation from the ideas in the culture at large. A "whole network of interests" prevails in any time and place.[29] The link assumes that biblical interpretations participated in this common discourse, a "web" which continues to proliferate, innovate, and create further ways of structuring ideas on rape. Hence, the procedure places biblical interpretations into a fabric, so that the emerging ideas can be evaluated in relation to the broader discourse.

The analysis of contemporary biblical interpretations demonstrates that the twentieth-century discourse includes opposing ideas on rape. For example, several interpretations emphasize the male characters of Genesis 34 whereas feminist scholarship stresses the significance of

---

[28] Michel Foucault, *The History of Sexuality*, vol. 1: *An Introduction*, trans. Robert Hurley (New York, Random House, 1978).

[29] Edward W. Said, *Orientalism* (New York: Random House, 1978), 3.

raped victim-survivors. In contrast to the discourse on rape in nineteenth-century Germany, which appeared to be cohesive, the contemporary period reflects disjunction. The gap might relate to the power
discrepancy within contemporary discourse.[30] Feminist scholarship has
emerged from a political and social movement in the 1960s which
questioned the status quo. Often biblical scholars did not connect to
this critique and rejected the political implications of such a critique.
Often they have handed down pre-feminist views as exemplified by
nineteenth-century interpretations and textbooks. In the contemporary period opposing views are publicly articulated, and so the current
discourse on rape reflects this tension. The correlation of opposing
views shows the extent of the conflict. The exegesis of Genesis 34
favors a contemporary feminist perspective, and thus resolves the tension.

A Feminist Standpoint

"Starting thought from women's lives,"[31] feminist standpoint theorists
analyze the causes for women's conditions and debate how to change
those conditions in conjunction with other oppressive structures. The
theorists have contributed significantly to the epistemological discussion about the value of a feminist standpoint as opposed to claims of
objectivity or relativity. In an article about the need to locate feminist
analysis, Donna Haraway opposes claims of both objectivity and relativism.[32] She considers scholarship done from "nowhere" (objectivity)
and from "everywhere" (relativism) an illusion, a "god-trick." Similar
to objectivistic statements, relativistic statements are a "way of being
nowhere while claiming to be everywhere equally." As such, relativism
is "the perfect mirror twin of totalization in the ideologies of objectivity; both deny the stakes in location, embodiment, and partial per-

---

[30] On the issue of power in societies, cf. Foucault, *The History of Sexuality*, 73,
97.

[31] Sandra Harding, *Whose Science? Whose Knowledge? Thinking from Women's
Lives* (Ithaca, NY: Cornell University Press, 1991), 150. For a recent discussion
about feminist standpoint theory see Susan Hekman, "Truth and Method: Feminist
Standpoint Theory Revisited," *Signs* 22, no. 2 (Winter 1997): 341-65, and the included responses in the same volume.

[32] Donna J. Haraway, "Situated Knowledges: The Science Question in Feminism
and the Privilege of Partial Perspective," chap. in *Simians, Cyborgs, and Women:
The Reinvention of Nature* (New York: Routledge, 1991).

spective."[33] Relativism and objectivism are based on unlocatable knowledge claims; nobody can be called into account. Haraway criticizes this idea. She is joined by Susan Bordo, another feminist theorist: "One is always *somewhere*, and limited."[34] A feminist standpoint argues "for situated and embodied knowledge" and is "against various forms of unlocatable, and so irresponsible, knowledge claims."[35]

According to Haraway, the development of situated discourse is key to a feminist standpoint because interpretations from particular and specific locations promise "more adequate, sustained, objective, transforming accounts of the world."[36] Thus, a newly defined objectivity remains the goal. Such an objectivity recognizes partiality and limited locations. It is "a doctrine and practice . . . that privileges contestation, deconstruction, passionate construction, webbed connections, and hope for transformation of systems of knowledge and ways of seeing."[37] This definition originated with Sandra Harding, who distinguished among "value-free objectivity," "judgmental relativism," and "strong objectivity."[38] The first refers to arguments that presuppose one universally and eternally valid standard of judgment; the second that any judgment is equally valid; the third that all judgments are socially situated and require a critical evaluation to determine which social situations generate the most objective knowledge claims. The conscious choice of one's standpoint leads to the development of "strong objectivity," which can be defined as the recognition that all human knowledge is socially located.

Acknowledging the multitude of social locations does not mean, however, that all knowledge claims are equally valid. Haraway states that "the standpoints of the subjugated . . . are the preferred because in principle they are least likely to allow denial of the critical and interpretative core of all knowledge." In other words, the most objective

---

[33] Ibid., 191.

[34] Susan Bordo, "Feminism, Postmodernism, and Gender-Scepticism," in *Feminism/ Postmodernism*, ed. and with an introduction by Linda J. Nicholson (New York: Routledge, 1990), 145.

[35] Haraway, "Situated Knowledges," 191.

[36] Ibid.

[37] Ibid., 191f.

[38] Sandra Harding, *Whose Science? Whose Knowledge? Thinking from Women's Lives* (Ithaca, NY: Cornell University Press, 1991), 139.

knowledge claims derive from those who have the least interest in maintaining the status quo, those who are on the "other side."[39]

At the same time, subjugated standpoints should not be romanticized. It is not a simple task to "see from below." The standpoints of the subjugated require "critical examination, decoding, deconstruction, and interpretation" because they too are "not [an] 'innocent' position." Standpoints from below are preferred only because "the subjugated have a decent chance to be on to the god-trick and all its dazzling—and, therefore, blinding—illuminations."[40] At no time in history is a person able to be everything, and never is a person nobody. Scholarship from a subjugated standpoint is therefore "more adequate, sustained, objective" than scholarship that pretends to be objective or relative. Hence, a feminist standpoint aims to give "better accounts of the world."[41]

Drawing upon feminist standpoint theory, the following study analyzes Genesis 34 and selected interpretations from the perspective of the subjugated, the one who is raped rather than from the perspective of the powerful. Traditional interpretation derives from the perspective of the powerful. In contrast, the following analysis focuses on the phenomenon of rape and the woman Dinah as the victim and survivor. Literary critic Laura E. Tanner observed that the definition of the victim's experience as the reader's own not only questions "disembodied conventions of reading and criticism"[42] but "open[s] up avenues of imaginative opposition."[43] Although this study does not claim that the proposed feminist interpretation is the only plausible one, it presupposes with Haraway that some interpretations are worse accounts of the world.[44] If interpretations do not offer a critical reexami-

---

[39] Ibid., 150.

[40] All these quotes are from Haraway, "Situated Knowledges," 191.

[41] Ibid., 196.

[42] Laura E. Tanner, *Intimate Violence: Reading Rape and Torture in Twentieth-Century Fiction* (Bloomington: Indiana University Press, 1994), 35.

[43] Ibid., xiii.

[44] Haraway, "Situated Knowledges," 196: "The feminist standpoint theorists' goal . . . is better accounts of the world." Cf. also Robin Scroggs, "The Bible as Foundational Document," *Interpretation* 49, no. 1 (January 1995): 19, who observes: "If assessments about biblical faith and ethics are made from contemporary sensitivities about what is right or wrong, then it is our contemporary perspectives that are authoritative." For a view that collapses the meaning of the adjective "right" with "objective," see Mary Ann Tolbert, "Afterwords," 315: "A 'right' or 'objective' reading is finally impossible, for every reading will bear the stamp of the one who makes it."

nation but instead support or favor the status quo, they are "wrong." With such a presupposition the interpretation of biblical texts is political "because ways of understanding and representing the world are deployments of power or contestation of authority."[45]

Methodological Reasoning

The present study conveys an important methodological consequence that contradicts a principle ordinarily supported by biblical scholars. Often, biblical scholars who adhere to historical critical, anthropological-sociological, or literary methods are convinced that "exegesis" (i.e., a "reading out" of the text) is possible independently of one's location and convictions. Assuming that "reading out" of the text does not presuppose "reading in" the text (i.e., eisegesis), many academic readers of the Bible do not identify their interests and social location as crucial elements of their interpretations.[46] This view was already questioned in Plato's dialog *Theaetetus*. There Protagoras argued that "individual things are for me such as they appear to me, and for you in turn as they appear to you."[47] Twentieth-century philosophers have made major contributions toward this idea.[48] Feminist biblical scholarship and increasingly biblical cultural studies have built on it. For example, Fernando F. Segovia has claimed, "All exegesis is ultimately *eisegesis*," and Edward L. Greenstein wrote, "To engage in Biblical

---

[45] Paul B. Armstrong, *Conflicting Readings: Variety and Validity in Interpretation* (Chapel Hill: University of North Carolina Press, 1990), 134.

[46] Krister Stendhal argued for the differentiation between the historical analysis of texts and the search for a contemporary meaning, cf. his "Biblical Theology, Contemporary," *Interpreter's Dictionary of the Bible*, vol.1 (1962): 418-32. See also his SBL presidential address "The Bible as a Classic and the Bible as Holy Scripture," *Journal of Biblical Literature* 103, no. 1 (1984): 3-10.

[47] G. P. Goold, ed., *Theaetetus: Plato*, trans. H. North Fowler (Cambridge, MA: Harvard University Press, 1921), 152a.

[48] See, for example, Hans-Georg Gadamer, *Truth and Method* (New York: Seabury Press, 1975); Richard Rorty, *Philosophy and the Mirror of Nature* (Princeton: Princeton University Press, 1979). See, e.g., the recent evaluative essay by Jean Grondin, "Hermeneutics and Relativism," in *Festivals of Interpretation: Essays on Hans-Georg Gadamer's Work*, ed. Kathleen Wright (Albany: State University of New York Press, 1990), 42-62.

Criticism means we must exercise our beliefs."[49] In accordance with this critique my study demonstrates that historical critical, anthropological-sociological, or literary approaches engage in a "reading into" the text with or without the recognition of a reader.

Of the many works that have been influential in the conceptualization of the present case study on the discourse on rape in biblical scholarship, six publications from secular disciplines and four from religious-theological disciplines are especially important.[50] Methodologically, the representative studies use intertextual reading strategies and argue for contextualized analyses. The selection of these studies does not assume that other works do not proceed similarly. On the contrary, the academic discourse abounds with such studies. The small selection here attests to the validity of an intertextual and contextualized examination of biblical interpretations which is a primary concern of my work.

Secular Sources

First, the literary critic Kathryn Gravdal traced the development of representation and the cultural meaning of rape in medieval French literature. She integrated legal texts into literary analysis as it is done in the "law and literature movement."[51] Moving beyond the conventional boundaries of her discipline, Gravdal examined poetry, church documents, and medieval legal texts.[52] Her work inspired my research, in which forensic medical textbooks of nineteenth-century Germany constitute the cultural context for the study of biblical commentaries.

Second, in her dissertation *Was It Rape? Sexual Violence and the Construction of Gender in Legal-Medical and Literary Discourse (1770-1810)*, Alexa Thorisch-Larson provided evidence that legal judg-

---

[49] Fernando F. Segovia, "Cultural Studies and Contemporary Biblical Criticism: Ideological Criticism as Mode of Discourse," chap. in *Reading from This Place*, vol. 2, p. 16; Edward L. Greenstein, "Theory and Argument in Biblical Criticism," chap. in *Essays on Biblical Method and Translation*, Brown Judaism Studies 92 (Atlanta: Scholars Press, 1989), 68.

[50] For a general introduction to intertextuality see Barbara Godard, "Intertextuality," in *Encyclopedia of Contemporary Literary Theory: Approaches, Scholars, Terms*, ed. Irena R. Makaryk (Toronto: University of Toronto Press, 1993), 568-72.

[51] For a further discussion of this movement see Kathryn Gravdal, *Ravishing Maidens: Writing Rape in Medieval French Literature and Law* (Philadelphia: University of Pennsylvania Press, 1991), 16, 149, footnotes 52-54.

[52] Ibid.

ments about rape are linked to the literary production of the eighteenth and early nineteenth centuries in Germany.[53] Her examination of forensic medical cases and German literature indicated that the juxtaposition of forensic medical textbooks and biblical commentaries of nineteenth-century Germany can create a valid cultural connection between those different types of literature.

Third, Lynn Higgins and Brenda R. Silver offered a convincing rationale for integrating readings of literary and nonliterary texts. In their introduction to *Rape and Representation* they argued for "the complex intersection of rape and representation."[54] They described the term "representation" as cutting across "boundaries of juridical, diplomatic, political, and literary discourse."[55] When the different disciplines are read together, they yield a full picture of rape within a specific period. Similarly, my study crosses disciplinary boundaries by relating biblical interpretations to forensic medical textbooks and feminist scholarship.

Fourth, Andrea Freud Loewenstein examined how the personal-psychological lives of three gentile male novelists of the twentieth century shape the representation of Jews and women in their work.[56] Grounding her study in poststructuralist discourse, "whose focus is the examination of the Other,"[57] Loewenstein stated that she "began to explore the history of the Jews in England in an effort to place the literature I was reading for this study in a historical context."[58] She established the historical and literary context of the conscious and unconscious attitudes of these three writers toward one particular topic. Likewise, my study places biblical interpretations within the cultural context of forensic medicine and feminist scholarship and focuses on the topic of rape.

Fifth, in *Culture and Imperialism* Edward Said studied English and French novels since the nineteenth century in connection with

---

[53] Alexa Kay Larson-Thorisch, "Was It Rape? Sexual Violence and the Construction of Gender in Legal-Medical and Literary Discourse (1770-1810)" (Ph.D. diss., University of Wisconsin-Madison, 1994).

[54] Higgins and Silver, *Rape and Representation*.

[55] Ibid., 1.

[56] Andrea Freud Loewenstein, *Loathsome Jews and Engulfing Women: Metaphors of Projection in the Works of Wyndham Lewis, Charles Williams, and Graham Greene* (New York: New York University Press, 1993).

[57] Ibid., 70.

[58] Ibid., 17.

literature, historiography, philology, sociology, and literary history to disclose imperialist attitudes in these novels. Intertextual reading strategies traced the connection between practices such as slavery, colonialism, and racism, on the one hand, and literary productions such as novels, poetry, and philosophy, on the other hand. Comparing and contrasting different types of literature deepened the analysis.[59] Earlier, Said showed the link between the theory of a discourse such as Orientalism and social and political struggles.[60] In the earlier study he also combined different types of literature from various academic disciplines to characterize the Western image of the Orient as a scholarly construction. Similarly, this work on Genesis 34 compares and contrasts different types of literature to uncover the ideas on rape as a scholarly construction connected to the practice of rape.

Sixth, in *Sociology and the Race Problem: The Failure of a Perspective* James B. McKee examined attitudes about race since the 1920s in sociology departments of American universities. By focusing on the failure of sociology to predict the black rebellion of the 1960s, he connected this discipline with events that occurred within society. He based the connection on the argument that "any act of textual interpretation must also recognize that the perspective being interpreted is embedded in a social context."[61] My case study similarly juxtaposes biblical interpretations with ideas from a cultural context, i.e., feminist scholarship, to understand and to evaluate the views of scholarly readers within a chosen context.

Religious-Theological Sources

Besides these publications from secular university settings, four studies from biblical scholarship and Christian theology have been crucial in developing this study. First, George Aichele and Gary A. Philips edited a collection of essays and claim in the introduction that "intertextuality has emerged as a fertile concept" in biblical scholarship. Intertextuality "serves as a critical gateway that opens out onto matters of ideology, subjectivity, the material production of meaning, and accountability."[62] Traditional boundaries of biblical scholarship

---

[59] Edward W. Said, *Culture and Imperialism* (New York: Knopf, 1993), xii-xiv.

[60] Said, *Orientalism.*

[61] James B. McKee, *Sociology and the Race Problem: The Failure of a Perspective* (Chicago: University of Illinois Press, 1993), 3

[62] George Aichele and Gary A. Philips, "Introduction: Exegesis, Eisegesis, Intergesis," *Semeia: Intertextuality and the Bible* 69/70 (1995), 7.

become obsolete because the understanding of "what is inside and what is outside" changes. Hence, "the rigid dichotomy between exegesis and eisegesis, between text and reading, between author and text, between text and reader"[63] loosens. Aichele and Phillips emphasized the significance of this change for biblical scholarship: "Meaning can no longer be thought of as an objective relation between text and extratextual reality, but instead it arises from the subjective, or ideological, juxtaposing of text with text *on behalf of* specific readers in specific historical/material situations in order to produce new constellations of texts/readers/readings."[64] Overall, the collection of essays exemplified the meaning of intertextuality for biblical scholarship, a meaning that the analysis of interpretations on Genesis 34 also explicates. Readers, their interpretations, and the question about their interests become central.

Second, in the collection entitled *Reading between Texts: Intertextuality and the Hebrew Bible*, the editor Danna Nolan Fewell maintained that "no text exists in a vacuum" but a text belongs to a larger "web" of texts.[65] Although the volume applied intertextual reading strategies only to interpret one biblical text in conjunction with another, the volume belonged to the larger endeavor of examining biblical interpretations in an interdisciplinary way. The latter endeavor characterizes this study.

Third, two recent volumes edited by biblical scholars Fernando F. Segovia and Mary Ann Tolbert supported the task of contextualizing biblical scholarship.[66] Focused on the "social location" of biblical texts and readers, the two volumes of *Reading from This Place* stressed the necessity of examining the context of interpretations by employing intertextual reading strategies. The key question to be asked in every reading is, "Whose meaning and whose truth?"[67] The following chapters keep this question present in the analysis of interpretations from the nineteenth and twentieth centuries.

Fourth, Mary McClintock Fulkerson, a feminist theologian, proposes in *Changing the Subject: Women's Discourses and Feminist Theol-*

---

[63] Ibid., 14.

[64] Ibid., 15.

[65] Danna Nolan Fewell, ed., *Reading between Texts: Intertextuality and the Hebrew Bible* (Louisville, KY: Westminster/Knox Press, 1992), 17.

[66] Segovia and Tolbert, eds., *Reading from This Place.*

[67] Gale A. Yee, "The Author/Text/Reader and Power: Suggestions for a Critical Framework for Biblical Studies," in *Reading from This Place*, vol. 1, 118.

ogy that boundaries of interpretation must be redrawn in a postmodern cultural reading of biblical texts. Removing neither text nor interpreter, the goal is "to see how larger domains of discourse and of social location bring them into being."[68] She applied intertextual reading strategies to both written texts and to cultural and social realities, such as—in the particularities of her study—oral interpretive traditions in churches, call stories, worship practices and performances. Meaning emerges from the juxtaposition of differently located "texts."[69] My case study appropriates the insight.

All these works from secular and religious-theological sources provide conceptual legitimacy for the procedure applied in the following chapters: using intertextual reading strategies to analyze biblical scholarship in correlation to a selected cultural perspective. Such an analysis cannot be done from a neutral or distanced perspective. Here the chosen "politics of location" is a feminist standpoint.[70]

---

[68] Mary McClintock Fulkerson, *Changing the Subject: Women's Discourse and Feminist Theology* (Minneapolis: Fortress, 1994), 144.

[69] Ibid., 165. "Text" is not limited to what is written. Fulkerson stated on p. 165: "The notion of textuality serves as a metaphor for cultural and social realities as well as written texts."

[70] Mary Ann Tolbert, "Afterwords: The Politics of Location," in *Reading from This Place*, vol. 2, 311.

Chapter 2

Defining Rape:
Feminist Scholarship on Rape
since the 1970s

Feminists from all over the world have extensively studied rape and have questioned long-standing assumptions and biases about rape. Scholarship on the subject has proliferated, emerging from various disciplines. Scholars have studied the experience from the perspective of the victim-survivors and helped trace the origin, causes, and reasons for the contemporary prevalence of rape. This chapter presents the development and discusses major concepts of the feminist discourse. It serves as the cultural context for the analysis of the biblical and forensic medical literatures.

Two sections organize the discussion. The first describes epistemological premises for theorizing about rape. The second section, the core of the chapter, discusses ideas about rape.

The Epistemology of Rape

In the 1970s most feminist analyses relied on the foundational premise that biological sex differences lead to the increasing prevalence of rape. Susan Brownmiller stated in her pioneering work that "we cannot work around the fact that in terms of human anatomy the possibility of forcible intercourse incontrovertibly exists. This single factor may have been sufficient to have caused the creation of a male ideology of rape."[1] In prehistoric times men discovered their genitalia as "weap-

---

[1] Susan Brownmiller, *Against Our Will: Men, Women and Rape* (New York: Bantam, 1975), 4.

ons," "along with the use of fire and the first crude stone axe."[2] For Brownmiller rape is part of the male biological predisposition and hence part of human history. Her study presents that history, premising "man's structural capacity to rape and women's corresponding structural vulnerability . . . as basic to the physiology of both our sexes."[3]

Postmodern feminists have criticized this pioneering study as an example of an essentialist, ahistorical, and universal analysis.[4] They challenge the assumption that biology is a "given reality," preceding social construction of "man" and "woman." In their view gender and sex have no preexisting basis. They do not consider the categories "woman" and "man" to be self-explicatory and self-sufficient. Rather, these categories are themselves "in process, a becoming, a constructing that cannot rightfully be said to originate or to end."[5] Over against Brownmiller they reject biologically based discussions of rape. In their place they put historically specific analyses based on the premise that all knowledge is constructed.[6]

---

[2] Ibid., 5.

[3] Ibid., 4.

[4] For postmodern feminism see Judith Butler, *Gender Trouble: Feminism and the Subversion of Identity* (New York: Routledge, 1990); ibid., "Imitation and Gender Insubordination," in *inside/out: Lesbian Theories, Gay Theories*, ed. Diana Fuss (New York: Routledge, 1991), 13-31; Patricia Hill Collins, *Black Feminist Thought: Knowledge, Consciousness, and the Politics of Empowerment* (New York: Routledge, 1990); Sandra Harding, "The Instability of the Analytical Categories of Feminist Theory," *Signs* 11, no. 4 (1986): 645-64; bell hooks, *Yearning: Race, Gender, and Cultural Politics* (Boston: South End Press, 1990); Stanlie M. James and Abena P. A. Busia, eds., *Theorizing Black Feminisms: The Visionary Pragmatism of Black Women* (New York: Routledge, 1993); Chandry Talpade Mohanty, "Under Western Eyes: Feminist Scholarship and Colonial Discourses," in *Third World Women and the Politics of Feminism*, ed. Ch. T. Mohanty, Ann Russo, and Lourdes Torres (Bloomington: Indiana University Press, 1991); Linda J. Nicholson, *Feminism/ Postmodernism* (New York: Routledge, 1990); Carol Smart, *Law, Crime and Sexuality: Essays in Feminism* (London: Sage, 1995); Elizabeth V. Spelman, *Inessential Women: Problems of Exclusion in Feminist Thought* (Boston: Beacon, 1988).

[5] Butler, *Gender Trouble*, 33.

[6] Scholars debated this point since Plato who claimed that the signified precedes the signifier. The basic difference between the early and the postmodern position on rape may finally be unresolvable. For a brief overview of Plato's ideas see, for example, *The Oxford Companion to Philosophy*, 1995 ed., under "Cave, analogy of," "Forms, Platonic," and "Plato." For a classic treatment of this foundational debate see David Ross, *Plato's Theory of Ideas* (Oxford: Oxford University Press, 1951), esp. 69-77.

But as a result, postmodern feminists often have not engaged the topic of rape. The omission has led Mary E. Hawkesworth to criticize postmodern feminism.[7] Considering herself a postmodern feminist who values the claims that all knowledge is mediated, that no naked facts await discovery, and that discourse itself, rather than a preexisting reality, creates "woman," Hawkesworth criticizes postmodern feminists for abstaining from discussions about rape, even though it belongs to the "few realities that circumscribe women's lives." Trapped in theory, the discussions fail to turn to specific problems that constitute a major problem in the lives of many women. As a result, postmodern feminists have not offered "crucial social and political insights" regarding rape.[8]

Sharon Marcus finds inconsistency in Hawkesworth's position, based on the fallacy of essentialism. She writes, "To treat rape simply as one of what Hawkesworth calls 'the realities that circumscribe women's lives' can mean to consider rape as terrifyingly unnameable and unrepresentable, a reality that lies beyond our grasp and which we can only experience as grasping and encircling us." Rape appears as a "fate worse than, or tantamount to, death."[9] By contrast, Marcus works toward an analysis that premises the possibility of ending rape. Working with the postmodern insight that no prior reality precedes language,[10] she proposes to treat rape as a "linguistic fact: to ask how the violence of rape is enabled by narratives, complexes, and institutions

---

[7] Mary E. Hawkesworth, "Knowers, Knowing, Known: Feminist Theory and Claims of Truth," *Signs* 14, no. 3 (1989): 533-57.

[8] Ibid., 555. Postmodern feminists are often criticized for lacking political vision. For a recent debate on feminist postmodernism see Joan Hoff, "Gender as a Postmodern Category of Paralysis," *Women's History Review* 3 (1994): 149-68; Susan Kingsley Kent, "Mistrials and Diatribulations: A Reply to Joan Hoff," *Women's History Review* 5, no. 1 (1996): 9-18; Caroline Ramazanoglu, "Unravelling Postmodern Paralysis: A Response to Joan Hoff," *Women's History Review* 5, no. 1 (1996): 19-23; Joan Hoff, "A Reply to My Critics," *Women's History Review* 5, no. 1 (1996): 25-30.

[9] Sharon Marcus, "Fighting Bodies, Fighting Words: A Theory and Politics of Rape Prevention," in *Feminists Theorize the Political*, ed. Judith Butler and Joan W. Scott (New York: Routledge, 1992), 387.

[10] For a clear and brief summary on postmodernism see Rachel T. Hare-Mustin and Jeanne Marecek, "Gender and the Meaning of Difference: Postmodernism and Psychology," in *Making a Difference: Psychology and the Construction of Gender*, ed. Rachel T. Hare-Mustin and Jeanne Marecek (New Haven, CT: Yale University Press, 1990), 24-27. See also Carol Smart, "Law, Feminism and Sexuality: From Essence to Ethics?" chap. in *Law, Crime and Sexuality: Essays in Feminism* (London: Sage, 1995).

which derive their strength not from outright, immutable, unbeatable force but rather from their power to structure our lives as imposing cultural scripts. Understanding rape as linguistically defined would understand it as subject to change."[11] This view enables Marcus to challenge the prevalence of rape from a theoretical perspective and to control a situation which seems to worsen continuously.

Marcus stresses the fact that, what she calls the "rape script" relies on conventional patterns of masculinity and femininity. Analysis has to uncover that, in this "gendered grammar of violence,"[12] men are the agents of violence and women are the subjects of fear. The pattern can only be fought by "putting into place what the rape script stultifies and excludes—women's will, agency, and capacity for violence."[13] Thus, women have to resist the rapist and recognize their own power to do violence so that theory will not consign them to biological weakness. Marcus's views contain liberating power because they see the "rape script" as changeable. To examine these scripts is one way "to frighten rape culture to death."[14] Andrea Benton Rushing agrees that such an analysis would invite a "politics of rape prevention"[15] instead of continuously refining the "treatment of the inevitable" without a "plan to end rape."[16]

Although it is true that postmodern feminists have not concentrated on rape,[17] they have contributed the epistemological insight that rape has to be theorized as a cultural construct. Discourse about it should not be based on foundationalist, preexisting concepts. Rape must be

---

[11] Marcus, "Fighting Bodies," 388f.

[12] Ibid., 393.

[13] Ibid., 395. For an analysis of rape scripts from a psychological perspective see Kathryn M. Ryan, "Rape and Seduction Scripts," *Psychology of Women Quarterly* 12 (1988): 237-45.

[14] Marcus, "Fighting Bodies," 401.

[15] Ibid., 386.

[16] Andrea Benton Rushing, "Surviving Rape: A Morning/Mourning Ritual," in *Theorizing Black Feminisms: The Visionary Pragmatism of Black Women*, ed. Stanlie M. James and Abena P. A. Busia (New York: Routledge, 1993), 130.

[17] For arguments in addition to those of Hawkesworth see Smart, *Law, Crime and Sexuality*, 109; for a critique of a postmodern evaluation of rape see Monique Plaza, "Our Damages and Their Compensation: Rape: The Will Not to Know of Michel Foucault," *Feminist Issues* (Summer 1981), 25-35; Teresa de Lauretis, "Violence of Rhetoric: Considerations on Representation and Gender," chap. in *Technologies of Gender: Essays on Theory, Film, and Fiction* (Bloomington: Indiana University Press, 1987).

understood as "culturally produced *at every level*."[18] Common cultural scripts, not the biological constitution of women, define women as objects for rape. The seemingly omnipresent existence of rape has to be understood in historical, particular, and specific terms, so that the situation can be changed. The examination of these scripts empowers women because it breaks prescribed patterns and constructs a vision of "a world free of rape."[19]

Feminist Ideas on Rape

The literature on rape is so extensive that any discussion must remain incomplete. From the plethora of scholarship five topics report on major developments and concepts.

Rape: Issues of Violence and Sexuality

Understanding rape in relation to violence and sexuality has developed in three stages: rape as biological expression of violence; rape as societal expression of violence; and rape as sexual violence.

Biological Expression

The pioneer effort of Susan Brownmiller on the subject of rape has already been acknowledged. The intent here is to explore further her ideas and then to present criticism of them. Considering rape as an act of violence, Brownmiller grounded her analysis in biology. Because of the "accident of biology," human anatomy brought "forcible intercourse incontrovertibly" into existence.[20] "Male nature" created rape to keep "*all women* in a state of fear."[21] Twelve chapters describe the history of rape, emphasizing American and Western history. Biblical references and examples from non-Western countries such as Bangladesh and the Congo are interspersed. At the end of the book Brownmiller offers consolation to women: They can fight back and defend themselves from their attackers by exploiting the "anatomical fact that the male sex organ . . . [has] at its root an awkward place of

---

[18] Winifred Woodhull, "Sexuality, Power, and the Question of Rape," in *Feminism and Foucault: Reflections on Resistance*, ed. Irene Diamond and Lee Quinby (Boston: Northeastern University Press, 1988), 174.

[19] Rus Erwin Funk, *Stopping Rape: A Challenge for Men* (Philadelphia: New Society, 1993), 153.

[20] Brownmiller, *Against Our Will*, 4.

[21] Ibid., 5.

painful vulnerability." Women should "make full use of a natural advantage . . . couched in phrases like emasculation, castration and ball-
breaking."[22] After all, men also have "that very special physical vulnerability."[23]

Brownmiller's work has been criticized by several scholars, such as
Catherine MacKinnon who rejects biology as an explanation for rape.
She contends that *biological* differences between women and men do
not account for the *social* oppression of women. She opposes the
view that inequality between women and men is the result of biological differences as tantamount to conceding that "biology is destiny."
Opposing such "feminist naturalism," she sees rape as an expression
of sexuality, "the dynamic of control by which male dominance . . .
eroticizes and thus defines man and woman, gender identity and sexual
pleasure."[24] According to MacKinnon, sexuality is "the experience of
power in its gendered form,"[25] so that "sexuality is violent" and "violence is sexual."[26] Rape has to be understood as a societal problem,
not as a "biologically inevitable"[27] phenomenon.

Jacquelyn Dowd Hall is another critic. She recognizes Brownmiller's
work as "an important milestone"[28] but criticizes her universalizing
and timeless view of rape. Hall argues for a specific and particular
historical examination in which Brownmiller would have addressed
the collaboration of women and their sources of power. She presents
a comparative example. Black Americans lacked economic support
and independence when they gained political rights after the Civil
War. As a result, they suffered persecution by lynching. Similarly,
women have asserted their rights since the 1970s without achieving
economic independence from men. Since that time women have suffered from rape in increasing numbers.[29] Such an analogy between

---

[22] Ibid., 454.

[23] Ibid.

[24] Catherine A. MacKinnon, *Toward a Feminist Theory of the State* (Cambridge,
MA: Harvard University Press, 1989), 137.

[25] Ibid., xiii.

[26] Ibid., 179.

[27] Ibid, 57.

[28] Jacquelyn Dowd Hall, "'The Mind That Burns in Each Body': Women, Rape,
and Racial Violence," in *Powers of Desire: The Politics of Sexuality*, ed. Ann Snitow,
Christine Stansell, and Sharon Thompson (New York: Monthly Review Press, 1983),
341.

[29] Ibid., 344.

rape and lynching demonstrates for Hall that the historical analysis of the oppression of people contributes to the understanding of rape in a way that biological explanations cannot. Hence, any rape analysis "must make clear its stand against *all* uses of violence for the purpose of oppression."[30]

Yet another critic is Bettina Aptheker who shows the complexities of the situation in her criticism of Brownmiller. She agrees that "rape was a politically motivated act of violence against women." However, an analysis of this topic should be linked with the oppression of African American men and all women.[31] Although Brownmiller addressed the issue of rape and racism in a chapter, Aptheker thinks that the "chasm of history" prevented her from taking a point of view "in which lynching and rape could be seen as *equally* atrocious and politically *connected* acts of terror."[32] She criticizes Brownmiller for elevating rape over other atrocities.

Societal Expression

In the landmark essay, "Rape: The All-American Crime," published in 1971, Susan Griffin defines rape as "a form of mass terrorism," "an act of aggression" and "violence." As a tool of "white male hierarchy," rape is "a classic act of domination," an expression of a power structure which not only "victimizes women" but engages in "raping Black people and the very earth we live upon."[33] Rape connects to all forms of violent oppression in the world; it exemplifies unjust hierarchical structures that go beyond gender relations.

From an anthropological perspective Peggy Reeves Sanday differentiates between "rape-free" and "rape-prone" societies to demonstrate that societal aggression, not biological differences between women and men, is the foundation of rape. In the context of the United States, she describes the connection of rape and the sexual aggression of young men at universities. According to her study, the privileged male status—dominant in American society—causes rape. By raping women, men keep women in a hierarchically lower place,

---

[30] Ibid., 346.

[31] Bettina Aptheker, *Woman's Legacy: Essays on Race, Sex, and Class in American History* (Amherst: University of Massachusetts Press, 1982), 53. This quote shows that Aptheker did not consider rapes committed by black men.

[32] Ibid., 54.

[33] Susan Griffin, "Rape: The All-American Crime," *Ramparts* (1971): 35.

the defining characteristic of rape-prone societies.[34] Rape reflects the struggle for material resources and societal control in the face of difficult circumstances.

The voices of raped women contributed substantially to the concept of rape as societal violence. Diana E. H. Russell interviewed several women about their rape experiences.[35] Their responses show that women feel violated in their innermost being after a rape. The violation of the victim's personhood emerges as the core element. Fear, depression, and overall anxiety are dominant factors. Margaret T. Gordon and Stephanie Riger argue that most women in the United States fear rape, and so their lives become seriously limited.[36] The violence of rape keeps women in their societal place.

Sexual Violence

Yet another understanding of rape in relation to sex and violence stresses its similarity to everyday heterosexual behavior.[37] Pamela Foe argues that the worst aspect of rape is a function of its place in society's sexual views. She equates rape with active sexual contact because "we are taught sexual desires are desires women ought not to have and men must have." This teaching sets up the condition for "an eternal battle of the sexes."[38] Rape "makes evident the essentially sexual nature of women,"[39] so that women feel humiliated when raped. Only the clarification of "our deep confusion about the place of, and need for, sexual relationship and the role of pleasure and intimacy in those relationships" might create a "sexually healthier society."[40] In such a society "the pleasure of friendship" would overcome the current "rape model of sexuality."[41]

---

[34] Peggy Reeves Sanday, *Fraternity Gang Rape: Sex, Brotherhood, and Privilege on Campus* (New York: New York University Press, 1990); see also Peggy Reeves Sanday, "The Socio-Cultural Context of Rape," *Journal of Social Issues* 37, no. 4 (1981): 5-27.

[35] Diana E. H. Russell, *The Politics of Rape: The Victim's Perspective* (New York: Stein and Day, 1984).

[36] Margaret T. Gordon and Stephanie Riger, *The Female Fear* (New York: Free Press, 1989).

[37] Pamela Foe, "What's Wrong with Rape," in *Feminism and Philosophy*, ed. Mary Vetterling-Braggin, Frederick A. Elliston, and Jane English (Totowa, NJ: Littlefield, Adams, 1981), 347-59.

[38] Ibid., 357.

[39] Ibid., 352.

[40] Ibid., 354.

[41] Ibid., 357.

This view emerges from her work on feminist legal discourse. MacKinnon observes that raped women often report problems with heterosexual intercourse after the rape experience: "It was her sexuality that was violated."[42] For MacKinnon rape and heterosexuality are "mutually definitive rather than mutually exclusive;"[43] rape is understood as a part of heterosexuality. Since the interaction between men and women requires the presence of the active and the passive, the actor and the acted upon, the superior and the inferior, this system applies to both heterosexuality and rape. Therefore, "sexuality is violent" and "violence is sexual."[44] All heterosexuality becomes rape because heterosexuality contains the dynamic that is clearly recognizable in the violence of rape.[45] The violence of rape merges with heterosexuality. MacKinnon regards rape as not being outside the realm of everyday heterosexual behavior: Heterosexuality models rape.

Winifred Woodhull supports the view of rape as everyday sexual violence.[46] She proposes that the understanding of societal power dynamics has to integrate the analysis of rape. The social mechanism has to be decoded to uncover the connection between sexuality and power:

> If we are seriously to come to terms with rape, we must explain how the vagina comes to be coded—and experienced—as a place of emptiness and vulnerability, the penis as a weapon, and intercourse as violation, rather than naturalize these processes through references to "basic" physiology.[47]

The goal is to generate new concepts and to challenge "the principles and practices of the current social order," so that the destructive force of rape disappears and women are empowered.[48] Relying on the work of French philosopher Michel Foucault, Woodhull criticizes him on two accounts. First, Foucault defined rape

---

[42] Catherine MacKinnon, "Sex and Violence: A Perspective," in *Rape and Society*, 30.

[43] MacKinnon, *Feminist Theory*, 174; see also Gregory M. Matoesian, *Reproducing Rape: Domination through Talk in the Courtroom* (Chicago: University of Chicago Press, 1993).

[44] MacKinnon, *Feminist Theory*, 179.

[45] For an expanded treatment of this thesis see Andrea Dworkin, *Intercourse* (New York: Free Press, 1987).

[46] Woodhull, "Sexuality, Power, and the Question of Rape," 167-76.

[47] Ibid., 171.

[48] Ibid., 174.

as violence as if rape were unrelated to sexuality. Second, ignoring the impact of sexuality, he did not correlate rape with the power dynamics in society. Therefore, Woodhull asserts the need to theorize rape as sexual violence and to utilize it as a starting point for criticizing societal power dynamics.

The critique of rape as sexual violence within society finds support in the research of Liz Kelly.[49] Interviewing sixty women about their experience of rape, Kelly concludes that women do not experience an either or dichotomy between heterosexuality and rape but "a continuum moving from choice to pressure to coercion to force."[50] Kelly defines rape in a broad way, ranging from verbal harrassment and pressure to physical coercion and force. In fact, several women started defining some of their experiences as rape after they reflected on them during the interviews. Kelly states that "there is no clear distinction, therefore, between consensual sex and rape, but a continuum of pressure, threat, coercion and force."[51] The connection of rape and sexual behavior demonstrates that the Western gender hierarchy produces only a difference in degree, not in kind, between rape and heterosexuality. Rape questions the gender dynamic and emerges as a societally and culturally institutionalized expression of the violence present in this gender dynamic. The end of rape requires a change in understanding sexual behavior.[52]

Institutionalized Rape: The So-Called Second Assault

"I have had the misfortune of being raped twice—once in the park and again in the media," exclaimed a young woman in suing the journalist who reported her rape case. She argued, "When you are raped, who you are is totally meaningless, and that is what Mike McAlary did to me. It was as if he and his editors said: 'We are going to enact whatever we want on you, even lies, and it does not matter who you are or

---

[49] Liz Kelly, "The Continuum of Sexual Violence," in *Women, Violence and Social Control*, ed. Jalna Hanmer and Mary Maynard (Houndmills, UK: Macmillan, 1987), 46-60.

[50] Ibid., 54.

[51] Ibid., 58.

[52] See David Lisak, "Sexual Aggression, Masculinity, and Fathers," *Signs* 16 (Winter 1991): 238-62.

how you feel about it.' "[53] Rape is not only an individual attack against the body of the victim-survivor,[54] the attitude of society is equally destructive. Police, hospital personnel, the courts, counseling services, family members and friends, religious institutions, schools, the media, and even jokes all contribute to the continuous violation of the raped woman after the actual rape. The idea of the "second assault" conceptualizes rape as an institutionalized problem.

The early feminist work of Nancy Gager and Cathleen Schurr describes the institutionalization of rape by listing the ways in which police officers, medical providers, courtrooms, and counseling facilities contribute to the continuous discrimination against the victim-survivor.[55] When a raped woman faces the police, she often encounters distrust. Medical examination procedures violate her physical integrity. In the courtroom she is treated as if she were the accused. The authors see the solution to rape in creating a "more human society." Since this is a truly global aim, the analysis of Gager and Schurr is only a first step in the task.

Another early analysis of rape examines how the second assault contributes to the pervasiveness of rape in Western societies. Diana E. H. Russell scrutinizes the attitudes of psychiatrists and husbands,[56] who, because they often sympathize with the rapist, make the victim-survivor the guilty party. Lacking support and understanding, the raped

---

[53] Don Van Natta, "Facts, Lies and Opinions on Trial in Unusual Sidelight to Rape Case," *New York Times*, 29 January 1996, B1. As early as in 1983 journalists published guidelines about reporting on rape. See "Branch of National Union of Journalists Proposes Guidelines on Rape Reporting," *Media Report to Women* 11, no. 4 (July-August 1983): 3, 12, 13. See also Beth McGlashan, "Women Should Decide for Themselves If They Want Rape Known," *Media Report to Women* 10, no. 6 (June 1, 1982): 10-11.

[54] The expression attributes agency to the woman. "Victim-survivor" is preferable to "victim," which connotes passivity, and to "survivor," which makes the woman's innocence invisible.

[55] Nancy Gager and Cathleen Schurr, *Sexual Assault: Confronting Rape in America* (New York: Grosset & Dunlap, 1976). For a rather positive view of the police see William B. Sanders, *Rape and Woman's Identity* (Beverly Hills, CA: Sage, 1980). See also Rita Gunn and Candice Minch, "Unofficial and Offical Responses to Sexual Violence," *Resources for Feminist Research* 14 (December 1985-January 1986): 47-49.

[56] Russell, *Politics of Rape*, 221-30.

woman withdraws into silence. The recent study of Gregory M. Matoesian formulates the problem as follows:

> Far from being an isolated act committed by a few psychopathically deranged men, rape is a culturally conditioned and ideologically supported social fact, a form of social power sanctioned by the state and institutionalized into the structure of law and the legal system. The vast majority of rapes are, indeed, not violations but enforcements of the social order.[57]

Rape is socially enforced not only by the rapist but also by many institutions. Thus, reasons for rape go beyond individual psychopathologies; they are rooted in societal biases. In fewer than twenty-five years feminist scholarship has turned the argument about rape away from biology to society.

Various studies demonstrate the extent of this turn. They examine numerous academic disciplines—legal studies, political philosophy, psychology, biology, literary studies, and history—in regard to their positions on rape.[58] The studies provide insight about the prevalence of a "rape culture" in the Western hemisphere. They show that the "second assault" is not reducible to an individual police officer who mistreats a woman reporting a crime or a reporter writing about it; institutions as a whole contribute to the continuation and the prevalence of rape. This insight into "institutional rape" has invited discussions about the need of Western societies to submit to the less powerful. As put by Joyce E. Williams and Karen A. Holmes in their study on attitudes about rape among different American ethnic groups and social classes, it is "the system . . . which has institutionalized the powerlessness of women and minorities."[59]

---

[57] Gregory M. Matoesian, *Reproducing Rape: Domination through Talk in the Courtroom* (Chicago: University of Chicago Press, 1993).

[58] Sylvana Tomaselli and Roy Porter, *Rape* (New York: Basil Blackwell, 1986); Lynn A. Higgins and Brenda R. Silver, *Rape and Representation* (New York: Columbia University Press, 1991). For a critical assessment of psychological studies on rape see, for example, Florence L. Denmark and Susan B. Friedman, "Social Psychological Aspects of Rape," in *Violence against Women: A Critique of the Sociobiology of Rape*, ed. Suzanne R. Sunday and Ethel Tobach (New York: Gordian Press, 1985), 159-84; Colleen A. Ward, *Attitudes toward Rape: Feminist and Social Psychological Perspectives* (London: Sage, 1995).

[59] Joyce E. Williams and Karen A. Holmes, *The Second Assault: Rape and Public Attitudes* (Westport, CN: Greenwood, 1981), 190. The parallelization of "women and minorities" does only insufficiently reflect that many women belong to "minorities" in the United States and elsewhere. In addition, there are also black men who rape women. Some of the early work on the second assault did not adequately discuss these complexities.

Psychologically oriented research in particular has attempted to uncover attitudes about rape among the broader public. In the 1980s uncountable studies dealt with the problem of the societal disbelief and mistreatment of rape victim-survivors.[60] One study, conducted by Cheryl S. Alexander, examines how nurses perceive rape victims and comes to an intriguing conclusion. After questioning nurses about the degree to which they attribute responsibility to the raped woman compared with the victims of nonsexual crimes, Alexander shows that the attribution of responsibility depends on the general stance of a female nurse toward "societal rules and norms, her locus of control, and her perceptions of [her] own potential victimization."[61] The research suggests that someone who believes in the status quo of societal rules and norms will find it more difficult to trust the one who has been violated. Blaming the victim for the "failure" is the way out of the dilemma. By contrast, nurses who do not blame the raped woman show a general willingness to criticize societal structures. Alexander concludes that people who blame the raped victim-survivor support the status quo to prevent themselves from criticizing society. Their need to believe in a world where bad things do not happen to good people makes them blame the raped woman. The way people evaluate the victim-survivor is thus related to their general attitudes about society.

These attitudes are shaped, of course, in many different ways. One major factor in contemporary Western societies is the entertainment industry. Wayne Wilson demonstrates that rape movies have flourished since the invention of film making.[62] The early film *Blackmail*

---

[60] For a sample of these studies see Pauline B. Bart, "Rape as a Paradigm of Sexism in Society—Victimization and Its Discontents," *Women's Studies International Quarterly* 2 (1979): 347-357; Hubert S. Feild, "Attitudes toward Rape: A Comparative Analysis of Police, Rapists, Crisis Counselors, and Citizens," *Journal of Personality and Social Psychology* 36 (1978): 156-79; Bill Thornton and Richard M. Ryckman, "The Influence of a Rape Victim's Physical Attractiveness on Observers' Attributions of Responsibility," *Human Relations* 36, no. 6 (1983): 549-62; Nora K. Villemur and Janet Shibley Hude, "Effects of Sex of Defense Attorney, Sex of Juror, and Age and Attractiveness of the Victim on Mock Juror Decision Making in a Rape Case," *Sex Roles* 9, no. 9 (1983): 879-89; Joyce E. Williams, "Secondary Victimization: Confronting Public Attitudes about Rape," *Victimology: An International Journal* 9, no. 1 (1984): 66-81.

[61] Cheryl S. Alexander, "The Responsible Victim: Nurses' Perceptions of Victims of Rape," *Journal of Health and Social Behavior* 21, no. 1 (March 1980): 22-33.

[62] Wayne Wilson, "Rape as Entertainment," *Psychological Reports* 63 (1988): 607-10.

(1929) and more recent ones such as *Curtains* (1983) and *When She Says No* (1984) depict rape myths of the general public. Even jokes about rape reflect the continuous institutionalization of the phenomenon.[63] To deal with the pervasiveness of rape in contemporary society, Nancy Gamble and Lee Madigan suggest to utilize the concept of the second assault:

> We realized that the key to change for the rape survivor cannot be found in society at the present time. Society needs to validate the experience of the second rape to improve the rate of reporting and prosecuting. Until the second rape is stopped, little will be gained by changing any written laws pertaining to the first rape.[64]

The differentiation between the first and the second rape clarifies the multifaceted dimensions of rape. Rape is then not merely regarded as a misfortune for an individual woman or the brutal act of an individual rapist. Rather, it is understood as an expression of societal structures that support the violent denigration of women as a group.

The Problem of Acquaintance Rape

Although people imagine that rape involves a stranger hiding behind the bushes in a lonely field in the middle of the night and attacking a woman, most rapes occur between acquaintances. This insight into the prevalence of rape among nonstrangers has become increasingly recognized. In fact, acquaintance rape is the predominant form of rape in the United States. James D. Brewer argues that seventy-six percent of victim-survivors know their attackers. He suggests: "Wade out of the ankle-deep statistics and what you find is that we as a nation have a much bigger problem with acquaintance or nonstranger rape than we believed in the past."[65]

Researchers have conducted numerous studies to discover why the public perceives a victim-survivor of acquaintance rape less favorably than the victim-survivor of stranger rape. One study holds that the public considers the victim-survivor of acquaintance rape less trust-

---

[63] Jeffery L. Schrink, Eric D. Poole, and Robert M. Regoli, "Sexual Myths and Ridicule: A Content Analysis of Rape Jokes," *Psychology: A Quarterly Journal of Human Behavior* 19, no. 1 (1982): 1-6.

[64] Nancy L. Gamble and Lee Madigan, *The Second Rape: Society's Continued Betrayal of the Victim* (New York: Lexington, 1991).

[65] James D. Brewer, *The Danger from Strangers: Confronting the Threat of Assault* (New York: Plenum, 1994), 146.

worthy because she may have encouraged sexual intimacy. The opinion poll also shows that men and women judge the situation differently. Men perceive a victim-survivor less favorably than women. The evaluation also depends on the resistance the victim-survivor exercised, an ambiguous issue in many cases of acquaintance rape.[66] Judith Bridges and Christine A. McGrail maintain that the expectation of traditional sex roles significantly affect the evaluation of acquaintance rape. Expecting the female to set the limits during sexual interactions, people accuse the woman of failing to preserve the boundaries. The public attributes to a woman a bad reputation and finds her more promiscuous than the victim-survivor of stranger rape.[67]

Lois Pineau, a philosopher, asserts that especially in cases of acquaintance rape the wishes of the woman demand a clearer analysis than is currently available. Legal procedures should reflect this concern. Pineau wants the rapist to prove that he received an ongoing positive and encouraging response from the victim-survivor during sexual intimacy. Instead of focusing on the consent of the victim-survivor, the cross-examiner should ask the attacker for the reasons which made him assume mutual sexual enjoyment. This "communicative model of sexuality" allows the examiner "to discover how much respect there had been for the dialectics of desire."[68] Pineau imagines the examiner asking the accused:

> Did he ask her what she liked? If she was using contraceptives? If he should? What tone of voice did he use? How did she answer? Did she make any demands? Did she ask for penetration? How was that desire conveyed? Did he ever let up the pressure long enough to see if she was really that interested? Did he ask her which position she preferred?[69]

---

[66] James D. Johnson and Lee A. Jackson, "Assessing the Effects of Factors That Might Underlie the Differential Perception of Acquaintance and Stranger Rape," *Sex Roles* 19, no. 1-2 (1988): 37-45. For another study on the perception of acquaintance rape see Patricia A. Tetreault and Mark A. Barnett, "Reactions to Stranger and Acquaintance Rape," *Psychology of Women Quarterly* 11 (1987): 353-58.

[67] Judith S. Bridges and Christine A. McGrail, "Attributions of Responsibility for Date and Stranger Rape," *Sex Roles* 21, no. 3-4 (1989): 273-86. A similar description of the perception of acquaintance rape appears in James V. P. Check and Neil M. Malamuth, "Sex Role Stereotyping and Reactions to Depictions of Stranger Versus Acquaintance Rape," *Journal of Personality and Social Psychology* 45, No. 2 (1983): 344-56, esp. 353.

[68] Lois Pineau, "Date-Rape: A Feminist Analysis," *Law and Philosophy* 8, no. 2 (August 1989): 241.

[69] Ibid.

A focus on the attacker and his rationale for continuing to have intercourse would change the legal procedure because the "communicative nature of an encounter is much easier to establish than the occurrence of an episodic act of resistance."[70] This model offers an effective examination procedure, particularly in cases of acquaintance rape, in which physical injury or threat is rarely involved. In contrast to the dominant "aggressive-acquiescence" model, consent is no longer the issue; instead, one must ask why the rapist believed the sex was harmless.

Since acquaintance rape has become part of rape analysis, researchers have observed differences in cases of acquaintance rape. R. Lance Shotland distinguishes five types of acquaintance rape: "early date rape," "beginning date rape," "relational date rape," and "rape after a lasting, active sexual relationship *without* and *with* battery."[71] Although the classification is peculiar, for example, the differentiation between "early" and "beginning" date rape, he identifies different causes for each type of rape that are related psychologically to the rapist.

According to Shotland, men who commit early date rape—rape during the first date—have an "unrealistic" expectation about sex. In beginning date rape—rape after several dates—a man and a woman misperceive each other's sexual intentions. The man gets frustrated and angry, a situation that enhances the likelihood of rape. Relational date rape occurs when the rapist considers sex to be a sign of love. When the partner does not agree to have sex, anger and desire culminate in rape. The last two types of date rape describe the dynamic between sexually engaged couples. Shotland remarks that classic concepts such as the right of the husband to have sex with his wife lead to these types of rape. His research suggests that acquaintance rape is a profound problem of various origins, quantitatively more prevalent than stranger rape.

The law professor Susan Estrich provided the first comprehensive summary of the legal status of acquaintance rape in the United States.[72] She calls it "simple rape" according to terminology used in research of the 1960s.[73] Her analysis about the effects of law, judges, and jurors

---

[70] Ibid.

[71] R. Lance Shotland, "A Theory of the Causes of Courtship Rape: Part 2," *Journal of Social Issues* 48, no. 1 (1992): 127-43.

[72] Susan Estrich, *Real Rape* (Cambridge, MA: Harvard University Press, 1987).

[73] Harry Kalven and Hans Zeisel, *The American Jury* (Boston: Little, Brown, 1966).

shows that "simple rape is real rape."[74] Therefore, the concept of real
rape cannot be restricted to stranger rape as is commonly done.

Estrich illustrates the problem of acquaintance rape with an example from the Michigan courts in the 1980s. Struggling to expand
the definition of sexual intercourse, the reformers of legal statutes
faced two choices in designing the new law. On the one hand, the
new law could have been designed to side with the woman and ask the
court to trust the statement of a woman who claimed that she did not
consent to having sex. On the other hand, the new law could side with
the man by being based on a broad definition of force. Reformers
decided to focus on men, but the enacted law did not improve the
statistics or the assessment of prosecutors,[75] and accusations of acquaintance rape did become more credible. The laws themselves did
not lessen sufficiently incidences of acquaintance rape. Thus, Estrich
maintained: "Changing the words of statutes is not nearly so important as changing the way we understand them."[76] Then the time will
come "to announce to society our condemnation of simple rape."[77]

Not in Isolation: Rape, Race, Class, and Imperialism

Making Connections
"Feminist efforts to end male violence against women must be expanded into a movement to end all forms of violence,"[78] bell hooks
writes in 1984. Understanding rape as part of the broader pattern of
violence prevents a simplistic and dualistic explanation of rape. It is
not "men and patriarchy [that] are the sole evils," argues hooks, but
the "culture of violence" carried out through racism, classism, and
imperialism. hooks is tired of feminists who see women as innocent
victims of violence. She calls on women and men to acknowledge
their participation in creating a culture of violence. If feminists do not
adhere to a broader understanding of rape, they will continue to promote stereotypical ideas about women and men.

hooks urges feminists to consider rape in conjunction with race,
class, and imperialism so that rape does not emerge as the monolithic

---

[74] Estrich, *Real Rape*, 104.

[75] Ibid., 84-86.

[76] Ibid., 91.

[77] Ibid., 104.

[78] bell hooks, "Feminist Movement to End Violence," chap. in *Feminist Theory:
From Margin to Center* (Boston: South End, 1984), 130.

cause for the oppression of women. Earlier feminists were sometimes more ambiguous about this point. In 1971 Susan Griffin did connect rape with other forms of oppression, stating, "The same men and power structure who victimize women are engaged in the act of raping Vietnam, raping Black people and the very earth we live upon."[79] Rape and other forms of injustice are related in this sentence. However, three sentences later Griffin claims that "rape is the quintessential act of our civilization." Understood as the "quintessential act," rape attains a superior position, as if the previously made connections do not count. Sexism in the form of rape becomes the prime cause of oppression. This idea also emerges in interviews conducted by Russell with raped women from diverse backgrounds. Even though these women acknowledged other forms of oppression, sexism became for them the exclusive cause for rape.[80]

Lynn A. Curtis criticizes this tendency in early feminism by examining the connections between rape and race in the United States. She wonders "how rape by black men, especially on black women, is 'the symbolic expression of white male hierarchy.' "[81] She suggests that the analysis of rape has to include both sexism and racism to account more fully for the history of rape.

Angela Y. Davis also believes that "any attempt to treat it [rape] as an isolated phenomenon is bound to flounder,"[82] and considers rape within the framework of racism, classism, and imperialism. Drawing from American history, she examines the relationship between the crime of rape and the punishment of lynching in the South. Davis claims that the understanding of the phenomenon requires to connect the analysis of rape with the analysis of racism and the economic system. In this expanded purview, then, the meaning of rape cannot

---

[79] Griffin, "All-American Crime," 35.

[80] See the section "Rape and Race" in Russell, *The Politics of Rape*, 1975. For a critique of Russell see Angela Y. Davis, "Rape, Racism and the Capitalist Setting," *Black Scholar* 9, no. 7 (1978): 24-30, esp. 26-27.

[81] Lynn A. Curtis, "Rape, Race, and Culture: Some Speculations in Search of a Theory," in *Sexual Assault: The Victim and the Rapist*, ed. Marcia J. Walker and Stanley L. Brodsky (Toronto: Heath, 1976), 131.

[82] Angela Y. Davis, *Women, Race & Class* (New York: Random House, 1981), 201; see also Lynora Williams, "Violence against Women," *Black Scholar* 12, no. 1 (January-February 1981): 18-24; Jennifer Wriggins, "Rape, Racism, and the Law," in *Rape and Society: Readings on the Problem of Sexual Assault*, ed. Patricia Searles and Ronald J. Berger (Boulder, CO: Westview, 1995), 215-22.

be separated from racism and classism. Insisting on these connections, Davis brings her insight to the contemporary scene:

> The class structure of capitalism encourages men who wield power in the economic and political realm to become routine agents of sexual exploitation. The present rape epidemic occurs at a time when the capitalist class is furiously reasserting its authority in face of global and internal challenges. Both racism and sexism, central to its domestic strategy of increased economic exploitation, are receiving unprecedented encouragement. It is not a mere coincidence that as the incidence of rape has arisen, the position of women workers has visibly worsened. So severe are women's economic losses that their wages in relationship to men are lower than they were a decade ago. The proliferation of sexual violence is the brutal face of a generalized intensification of the sexism which necessarily accompanies this economic assault.[83]

For Davis the links among sexism, racism, and imperialism are key to understanding and stopping rape. The feminist author Jacqueline Hall agrees with Davis that the increasing number of rapes results from "women's economic vulnerability and relative powerlessness."[84] Analysis of rape has to connect to that of other forms of oppression.

Relating explanations of rape to other issues has a long history in the United States. Nineteenth-century African-American intellectuals such as Anna Julia H. Cooper, Ida B. Wells-Barnett, and Pauline E. Hopkins[85] linked the prevalence of rape not only to lynching but also to economic exploitation. The feminist scholar Hazel V. Carby summarizes their accomplishments: "Their analyses are dynamic and not limited to a parochial understanding of 'women's issues'; they have firmly established the dialectical relation between economic/political power and economic/sexual power in the battle for control of women's bodies."[86] Confronted with tremendous oppression, including rape,

---

[83] Davis, *Women, Race & Class*, 200.

[84] Jacqueline Dowd Hall, "The Mind That Burns in Each Body," 344.

[85] "Cooper, Anna Julia Haywood (1858-1964)," in *Black Women in America: An Historical Encyclopedia*, ed. Darlene Clark Hine, vol. 1 (Brooklyn, NY: Carlson, 1993), 275-81; "Wells-Barnett, Ida Bell (1862-1931)," in *Black Women in America*, vol. 2, 1242-1246; "Hopkins, Pauline Elizabeth (1859-1930)," in *Black Women in America*, vol. 1, 577-79.

[86] Hazel V. Carby, "'On the Threshold of Woman's Era': Lynching, Empire, and Sexuality in Black Feminist Theory," *Critical Inquiry* 12 (Autumn 1985): 276. For a study which focuses primarily on racism see Eric W. Rise, "Race, Rape, and Radicalism: The Case of the Martinsville Seven, 1949-1951," *Journal of Southern History* 58, no. 3 (August 1992): 461-90.

these intellectuals understood that an exclusive focus on rape is not sufficient to end the prevalence of rape. They recognized the need to combine the various forms of oppression of their time: rape, lynching, and economic exploitation. Rape was only one "weapon of terror of internal colonization."[87] Recognition of these connections helped them to find strategies for change.

A Missed Connection

A less successful example of historical research demonstrates by omission the importance of relating explanations of rape with different forms of oppression. The movie *BeFreier und Befreite* by the German filmmaker Helke Sander documents the huge numbers of rape committed on German women by Russian soldiers who occupied Berlin in May 1945.[88] Interviews show the effects of these rapes on the women. Publicly silenced after the war, they tell their stories in the documentary film more that forty years later, sometimes for the first time in their lives. The book, coproduced with the movie, includes references to official statistics on abortions and medical reports of venereal diseases, validating the women's experiences. Neither the film nor the book, however, explored the larger connection of women being raped by an offical enemy. Although the documentary takes the necessary step of reporting the rapes, the film does not analyze the implications of using rape as a tool for punishment. In addition, the interviews do not discuss the fact that the raped women were Germans who had lived under the Nazi regime and belonged to the nation that had lost the war. If the film had made these links, it might have opened a debate between nationalism and rape.

What Helke Sander failed to do for German women of the Nazi period, Darlene Clark Hine has done for nineteenth-century black women in the United States. She argues that black women developed "a cult of secrecy" as they faced the combined forces of racism, classism, sexism, and national economic differences. This "culture of dissem-

---

[87] Carby, "On the Threshold," 273.

[88] For their book see Helke Sander and Barbara Johr, eds., *BeFreier und Befreite: Krieg, Vergewaltigungen, Kinder* (Munich: Kunstmann, 1992). For a critique of the movie see Atina Grossmann, "A Question of Silence: The Rape of German Women by Occupation Soldiers," *October* 72 (Spring 1995): 43-63.

blance" helped them protect their inner lives.[89] The complex situation of German women who were raped in 1945 might have initiated a similar process of internal retreat and secrecy though for different reasons.[90]

Balancing Connections

Explanations of rape and analyses of other forms of oppression require balance—but as the anthropologist Diane Bell points out, these explanations must also not minimize the horror of the deed. While working with aboriginal women in Australia, Bell was accused of "imposing [her] agenda on other cultures."[91] Colleagues said that she ignored ethnic, racial, and cultural differences. Bell believes that her colleagues used these categories to silence her views. Insisting on the validity of gender analysis, she aims for a balance in discussing relations among gender, race, and violence. Not devaluing one issue for the other, she claims that her work serves the needs of aboriginal women. The validity of this claim appears in articles published by the aboriginal Topsy Napurrula Nelson who worked with Bell and participated with her in conferences. As a result, aboriginal women have become subjects of anthropological studies in which they previously were only objects. One significant issue in these studies is rape.

---

[89] Darlene Clark Hine, "Rape and the Inner Lives of Black Women in the Middle West," *Signs* 14, no. 4 (1989): 915. For a discussion of the "intersectionality" of analytic categories see Kimberlé Williams Crenshaw, "Mapping the Margins: Intersectionality, Identity Politics, and Violence against Women of Color," in *The Public Nature of Private Violence: The Discovery of Domestic Abuse*, ed. Martha Albertson Fineman and Roxanne Mykitiuk (New York: Routledge, 1994), 93-118.

[90] Perhaps in response to critiques of her work Sander plans to examine the consequences of German women's retreat into silence and to discuss that they were Germans raped by an enemy army. See Helke Sander and Roger Willemsen, *Gewaltakte, Männerphantasien & Krieg* (Hamburg: Ingrid Klein, 1993), 17, 100.

[91] Diane Bell, "Intraracial Rape Revisited: On Forging a Feminist Future beyond Factions and Frightening Politics," *Women's Studies International Forum* 14 (1991): 386. The recent debate about the rape of a twelve-year-old Japanese girl by three American soldiers demonstrates a similar problem. The rape inspired opposition to the American military occupation of the Japanese island of Okinawa. A full-page appeal by Japanese women's organizations in the *New York Times* on January 26, 1996, p. A13, implies that the American military is the only reason for rape in Japan. A more complex argument would consider the significance of the numerous Japanese rape comics, even for girls, as reported by the *New York Times* (November 5, 1995): D1, D6.

The reduction of rape to a woman's issue is another sign of lacking balance. It skews understanding the complex history of rape. In an essay on E. M. Forster's *A Passage to India*,[92] Jenny Sharpe maintains, for example, that exclusively anticolonialist or feminist interpretations have ignored the combined effect of racial and sexual assumptions in the novel. While the novel suggests an either or decision for the "English woman" or "the Indian man," such a separation serves the assumption that friendship between the colonized divide is impossible. Keeping the analysis of rape and racism together in the interpretation of the novel avoids a perspective that the colonizer constructed. When rape is seen within this complex situation, the issue belongs to more than women. It is a matter of global concern.

International Connections: Rape as a Global Problem

Feminists around the world have emphasized that rape is part of the larger issue of violence against women. The Fourth World Conference on Women held in Beijing in September 1995 demonstrated the global concern to eradicate such violence from the state, the community, and the individual. International connections broaden the perspective on rape beyond individual or psychological concerns. International debates support the earlier insight of Western feminists that rape is a worldwide problem.[93]

Most analyses from non-Western perspectives relate rape and violence against women to economic, political, and national situations. The South African Matlhogonolo Maboe reports that rape is closely linked to these factors. It hurts whole communities and reflects violence in the general society: "Women consider whatever happens to them as women in relation to their family, their violator, their community, as well as their religion, tradition, and culture."[94] Hence, an individual intervention process is not enough. Rape crisis programs have

---

[92] Jenny Sharpe, "The Unspeakable Limits of Rape: Colonial Violence and Counter-Insurgency," *Genders* 10 (Spring 1991): 25-46.

[93] Patricia D. Rozeé, "Forbidden or Forgiven? Rape in Cross-Cultural Perspective," *Psychology of Women Quarterly* 17 (1993): 499-514. For an Australian anthropological feminist perspective see also Diane Bell and Topsy Napurrula Nelson, "Speaking about Rape Is Everyone's Business," *Women's Studies International Forum* 12, no. 4 (1989): 403-16.

[94] Matlhogonolo Maboe, "Strategies to Tackle Rape and Violence against Women in South Africa," in *Gender Violence and Women's Human Rights in Africa*, ed. Center for Women's Global Leadership (Highland, NJ: Plowshares 1994), 30-37.

to be integrated into the larger communities. South African women created the "Men's Rape Awareness and Prevention groups."[95] Based on establishing connections among political, social, domestic, sexual, and state violence, programs deal with crisis, prevention, and support. They attempt to empower women. In addition to dealing with raped victim-survivors South African women use the issue of rape as the starting point for examining their "culture of violence."[96]

The feminist movement in India also understands rape as a form of injustice committed against women within a network of exploitative structures. In 1988, participants at a conference in Patna, India, concluded that "the challenge [is to give] a new, holistic but still materialistic explanation that can link together economic crises, ecological destruction, goondaizing [sic] trends in the State itself and the terrifying spasms of religious fundamentalism and communal violence, and define the ways these are associated with the victimization of women."[97] Indian feminists understand that rape enables the members of higher castes and classes to violate lower-caste and lower-class women. They categorized the subject into class rape, police rape, army rape, landlord rape, marital rape, rape within the family, and the rape of prostitutes. Rejecting "the patriarchal view of rape as a violation of honour,"[98] these feminists relate rape to other forms of societal ills. Gail Omvedt stresses that "questions of the interrelationship between violence, exploitation and sexuality . . . go to the heart of the question of violence against women."[99] A multifaceted issue, rape cannot easily be "healed." Society has to change.

The horror of rape during war was brought home recently by the rape of thousands of Bosnian women by Serbian soldiers.[100] These crimes, perpetrated on women of the besieged side by everyday soldiers, demonstrates that rape reaches beyond individual and psycho-

---

[95] Ibid., 34.

[96] Ibid., 36.

[97] Gail Omvedt, *Violence against Women: New Movements and New Theories in India* (New Delhi: Interpress, 1990), 4.

[98] Radha Kumar, "The Agitation against Rape," chap. in *The History of Doing: An Illustrated Account of Movements for Women's Rights and Feminism in India, 1800-1990* (London: Verso, 1993), 133.

[99] Ibid., 7. For an earlier report on rape in India see K. P. Krishna, "Rapes and Its Victims in India," *Journal of Social and Economic Studies* 10 (1982): 89-100.

[100] Amnesty International, *Bosnia-Herzegovina: Rape and Sexual Abuse by Armed Forces* (New York: Amnesty International, 1993).

logical explanations. Rape is a systematic method used by societies worldwide to dehumanize the victim-survivors.

Feminists from still other countries affirm the need to understand rape as a complex societal reality. Jane Held of Britain encourages the peace movement of her country to include the issue of violence against women in its agenda if it continues to claim that "peace is more than the absence of war."[101] Opal Palmer Adisa of the United States analyzes rape poems written by African-American women to show that rape is an international problem rooted in the complexities of economy and politics.[102] Women's voices from Zimbabwe and Malaysia likewise insist on the societal and economic dimensions of rape.[103] Internationalists at a conference in Jerusalem in 1986 reached similar conclusions.[104]

Aruna Gnanadason presents an impressive overview of different international voices, organizing against violence toward women.[105] She confirms that "the women's movement around the world has created the space and the environment in recent years for women to tell their stories of physical and mental intimidation, to speak out their pain to a world that must become aware of the propensity of the problem and must seek ways in which to respond."[106] The analysis of rape must include an analysis of the economic context and the dominant market paradigm which makes women vulnerable participants, particularly in countries where women are the sole household providers. Violence against women belongs to global structures of violence. For certain,

---

[101] Jane Held, "The British Peace Movement: A Critical Examination of Attitudes to Male Violence within the British Peace Movement, as Expressed with Regard to the 'Molesworth Rapes,'" *Women's Studies International Forum* 11, no. 3 (1988): 219.

[102] Opal Palmer Adisa, "Undeclared War: African-American Writers Explicating Rape," *Women's Studies International Forum* 15, no. 3 (1992): 363-74.

[103] A. Armstrong, *Women and Rape in Zimbabwe*, Human & People's Right Project, Monograph No. 10 (Lesotho: Institute of Southern African Studies, 1990); *Rape in Malaysia: The Victims and the Rapists: The Myths and the Realities: What Can Be Done* (Penang, Malaysia: Consumers' Association of Penang, 1988).

[104] Alison Solomon, "Congress on Rape: Jerusalem, April 7-10, 1986," *Women's Studies International Forum* 9, no. 3 (1986): i-iii.

[105] Aruna Gnanadason, "Violence against Women: Women against Violence," unpublished paper from a conference at the Rochester Divinity School, November 9-13, 1995.

[106] Ibid., 2.

ending rape and violence against women is an overwhelming task, huge in its scope.

Summary

The study, "Rape in America: A Report to the Nation," prepared by the National Victim Center in Arlington, Virginia, and the Crime Victims Research and Treatment Center in Charleston, South Carolina, states that 683,000 women are forcibly raped every year in the United States alone.[107] The number is low if one considers that the study applied the legal definition of rape or criminal sexual assault accepted by most American states. If the number of unreported or unrecognized rapes were taken into consideration, the statistic would be much higher. Rapes are epidemic and a reality in the lives of people during war and peace. Consequently, "There is no easy solution to preventing rape."[108] Hierarchy and submission define the interaction of women and men, as is reflected in economics, politics, and state relations.

Almost twenty years after Susan Griffin tried to "think of a world in which rape would be a foreign concept," it is still all too familiar. Her statement that "to dream of a world without rape is to dream of indeed a radically different world" remains valid for today.[109] Nevertheless, this overview demonstrates that feminist scholars have opened up new ways of thinking. A discourse rich in general and detailed ideas on rape has spread into academic disciplines over a wide spectrum. Science, psychology, sociology, political science, law, literature, history, biology, anthropology, and religious studies are among these disciplines.

Five topics have delineated major advances in feminist efforts to define rape. First, debates on biology have moved to questions of violence and sexuality. Whereas initially some feminists reduced rape to either of these issues, others have introduced the concept of sexual violence. Second, observations about institutional and societal support of rape myths and prejudices followed. Rape is now understood

---

[107] National Victim Center and Crime Victims Research and Treatment Center, *Rape in America: A Report to the Nation*, April 23, 1992.

[108] Julie A. Allison, *Rape: The Misunderstood Crime* (Newbury Park, CA: Sage, 1993), 151.

[109] Susan Griffin, "A History 1971-1978," chap. in *Rape: The Power of Consciousness* (New York: Harper & Row, 1979), 24f.

as a multifaceted concept. Numerous studies report the problem of the second assault often experienced by women who undergo medical treatment or court procedures. Laws have been criticized and changed; hospital treatments adapted to the needs of women. Other studies have discerned the second assault concept in literature, music, films, and even jokes. Third, stranger rape has been differentiated from acquaintance rape which itself takes various forms, such as early date rape, relational date rape, and marital rape. Fourth, feminist scholars have criticized the idea of sexism as the prime cause of rape and have shown that rape is connected to racism, classism, and imperialism. It is one expression of unjust, exploitative, and hierarchical societal structures. Fifth, the focus on rape as exclusively a woman's issue has become a global issue. International discussions about the prevalence of rape understands it as a phenomenon of violence.

In the following three chapters we will see that the discourse in biblical studies and forensic medicine in nineteenth-century Germany and the contemporary period did not emerge from a perspective sympathetic to the victim-survivors. On the contrary, researchers disqualified, distrusted, or ignored women's accounts. Participating in the institutionalization of rape, interpretations of Genesis 34 and forensic medical textbooks illustrate the thesis of feminist theorists that rape scripts enable the violence of rape. The next chapters exemplify the extent of such scripts that disregard the rape victim-survivor.

Chapter 3

Retrospecting Rape (Part One): Christian Commentaries on Genesis 34 in Nineteenth-Century Germany

Analyzing commentaries on Genesis 34 from nineteenth-century Germany demonstrates how biblical scholars of a specific time and place approached the issue of rape. I have been guided by four factors in choosing these commentaries. First, excelling during the nineteenth century, historical criticism proliferated and influenced several generations of biblical scholars. The disclosure of biases in interpretations of Genesis 34 from this period illuminates this heritage, which continues to affect contemporary interpretations. Second, commentaries represent a major tool in a theological library. Read not only by biblical scholars, they enjoy popularity among pastors, teachers, students, and laypeople. Third, German biblical studies have influenced biblical scholarship across the world. The commentaries under consideration offer pivotal samples to show the extent of that impact. Fourth, dealing with my own German and Christian theological heritage honors the current emphasis of working within one's own context.[1]

The analysis in this chapter confronts the commentaries with questions from a different and much later context. The commentators did not concentrate on the rape and often did not read Genesis 34 as a rape story. For purposes of this chapter the present analysis presup-

---

[1] A similar study could be done from numerous settings, such as Korean, Jewish-Israeli, Hispanic, French, British or American. For a summary of the history of Jewish interpretations of Genesis 34 see Naomi Graetz, "Dinah the Daughter," in *A Feminist Companion to Genesis*, ed. Athalia Brenner (Sheffield, UK: JSOT, 1993), 306-17.

poses Genesis 34 as a rape story and examines biblical interpretations in regard to their ideas on rape. The exegetical chapter will
present the argument behind this presupposition and show that the
rape is central to the narrative.

Historical Overview

During most of the nineteenth century, German Christian biblical scholars were divided into two camps: those who accepted and those who
rejected the discipline of historical criticism.[2] Commentaries on Genesis 34 reflected this polarization. Some commentators posed historical critical questions about the text, analyzing every biblical phrase
and verse to establish authorship and origin. Other commentators
wrote from the Confessional orthodox approach. Their interpretations conformed to the Augsburg Confession and presupposed "the
atoning work of Christ" as the starting point for reading the Bible in a
Christian manner. They maintained traditional views about authorship and origin.[3]

One of the most prominent opponents of historical criticism was
Ernst W. Hengstenberg. As a leading voice of Confessional orthodoxy, he successfully hindered the development of historical criticism
while he was a professor at the University of Berlin from 1828 to
1869. Hengstenberg's influence as a professor and established theologian dominated the middle forty years of the nineteenth century,[4]
including the incident that Hengstenberg never allowed the renowned
historical critical scholar Johann K. W. Vatke to become a full professor in Berlin.

Though Hengstenberg had many like-minded colleagues, some of
them, such as Franz Delitzsch, began to integrate historical criticism
into their work during the latter part of their careers. The various
editions of the Genesis commentary by Delitzsch reflected this development. In the second edition of 1853 Delitzsch stressed the fact that

---

[2] Though not considered here, Jewish biblical scholarship also flourished during
the nineteenth century in Germany. For a recent study of this area see Hans-Joachim
Bechtoldt, *Die jüdische Bibelkritik im 19. Jahrhundert* (Stuttgart: Kohlhammer, 1995).

[3] See John Rogerson, *Old Testament Criticism in the Nineteenth Century:
England and Germany* (London: Fortress, 1985), 79-90.

[4] Ibid., 85-90.

his interpretation presented the text "undivided."[5] Writing a commentary that "without divisions displays the living whole as alive,"[6] he did not allow the "critical element" to dominate. In fact, he harshly judged historical critical commentaries:

> Wenn man den kritischen, willkürlichen, exegetisch geistlosen Commentar über den Pentateuch von J. Severin Vater (3 th. 1802-05) und die scheinbar sehr gelehrte, aber liederliche und ungläubig freche Auslegung der Genesis von Peter v. Bohlen (1835) zusammennimmt, so wird man sich des Schmerzes über die Tiefe des Abfalls vom kirchlichen Schriftglauben nicht erwehren können. . . . Sie haben aber alle keinen Sinn für die heilige Schrift als ein Buch göttlicher Offenbarung, kein Interesse an dem Christenthum als Religion der Versöhnung und entziehen diesem deshalb mit einer tiefbetrübenden Gleichgültigkeit, die in Knobels Commentare ihren Tiefpunkt erreicht hat, ihre in der Genesis enthaltene und unveräusserliche urgeschichtliche Voraussetzung.[7]

> If one reads J. Severin Vater's (3 th. 1802-5) critical, arbitrary, exegetically spiritless commentary on the Pentateuch and Peter v. Bohlen's (1835) apparently learned but sloppy and extremely impudent interpretation of Genesis, one feels the pain about the depth of the decline from scriptural faith . . . . They all do not appreciate holy Scripture as a book of divine revelation and are not interested in Christianity as a religion of reconciliation. Therefore, with an indifference which culminates in Knobel's commentary and which is deeply saddening, they deprive Christianity of the inalienable prehistoric basis that is contained in Genesis.

Later, Delitzsch changed his stance. The fifth edition of his commentary included "preparatory works of Wellhausen, Kuenen and preferably Dillmann," though even then Delitzsch claimed that "the spirit of this commentary has remained the same since 1852,"[8] the year of

---

[5] Franz Delitzsch, *Die Genesis*, 2. umgearbeitete und erweiterte Auflage (Leipzig: Dörffling und Franke, 1853), vi.

[6] Ibid., vi: "welche das Ganze unzerstückt als lebendiges vorführt." For more information on the work of Delitzsch see Rogerson, *Old Testament Criticism*, 111-20; Hans-Joachim Kraus, *Geschichte der historischen-kritischen Erforschung des Alten Testaments*, 3. erweiterte Auflage (Neukirchen-Vluyn: Neukirchener, 1982), 230-41.

[7] Delitzsch, *Die Genesis*, 59f.

[8] Franz Delitzsch, *Neuer Commentar über die Genesis*, 5th ed. (Leipzig: Dörffling und Franke, 1887), iii. The translated commentary by Delitzsch, *A New Commentary on Genesis*, trans. Sophia Taylor, vol. I (New York: Scribner Welford, 1889), 23-28, supported historical critical scholarship and participated in historical critical discussions.

the first edition. Only after Hengstenberg's death did the "rational" historical critical approach to the Bible develop fully and with unobstructed force. The work of Julius Wellhausen represented this new space for historical criticism toward the end of the century.[9]

The commentaries on Genesis reflected the multifaceted attitudes toward historical criticism. Gottfried Hoberg devoted almost forty pages to explain its development.[10] Heinrich Holzinger presented a thorough description of the method.[11] Johann P. Lange questioned many historical critical insights; yet he also gave a long overview of the method.[12] Whether rejected, compromisingly tolerated, or accepted, historical criticism set the tone.

Interpretations of Genesis 34 also mirrored the debate. Some commentators were exclusively concerned with the linguistic history of this text so that they did not go beyond grammatical, stylistic, and comparative analyses. The commentaries of Bachmann, Kautzsch-Socin, Strack, and Vater belong into this category. Other commentaries combined discussions of historical criticism with questions about content. The commentaries of Delitzsch, Dillmann, Gunkel, and Tuch exemplified this combination. From the other side opponents of historical criticism wrote elaborate interpretations of Genesis 34 that went beyond the mere mechanical interests of certain historical critical scholars. Examples include the commentaries of the early Delitzsch, and of Baumgarten, Lange, and Thiersch. In most commentaries historical critical and Confessional approaches overlapped, and so they yielded discernible ideas about rape.

Ideas about Rape

Five ideas emerge. Some of them are explicitly stated; others require some explanation.

---

[9] Julius Wellhausen, *Prolegomena to the History of Ancient Israel* (New York: Meridian, 1957; first German ed. 1878). For further details see John Rogerson, *Old Testament Criticism*, 79-90, 257-89.

[10] Gottfried Hoberg, *Die Genesis nach dem Literalsinn erklärt* (Freiburg im Breisgau: Herder, 1899), xiii-xlix.

[11] Heinrich Holzinger, *Genesis, Kurzer Hand-Commentar zum Alten Testament* (Freiburg/Leipzig/Tübingen: J. C. B. Mohr, 1898), ix-xvi.

[12] Johann P. Lange, *Genesis or the First Book of Moses Together with a General Theological and Homiletical Introduction to the Old Testament*, trans. Taylor Lewis and A. Gosmann, 5th rev. ed. (New York: Scribner, 1884), 30-45. 94-99.

The Marginalization of Rape

Many commentaries on Genesis 34 barely mentioned rape. They mentioned it only in passing, and they focused on other topics. The choice of titles for issues discussed, the content of the interpretations, and the way in which Dinah was blamed all reflected the marginalization of the subject of rape.

Of twenty commentaries examined only four commentators referred to the rape in the titles that preface their discussion. Carl Friedrich Keil called this unit "Violation of Dinah, Revenge of Simeon and Levi— Chap. XXXIV."[13] Peter von Bohlen entitled his study "The Weakening of Dinah and the Massacre of Shechem."[14] August Dillmann chose "Jacob at Shechem and the Dishonoring of Dinah."[15] Hermann Strack combined two titles, one focusing on Jacob and another stressing the fraternal revenge: "Jacob at Shechem; Simeon and Levi Revenge the Dishonoring of Dinah."[16] Although the term "rape" was not used explicitly, the titles conceded that Dinah was somehow "violated."

Most titles did not mention the rape or indicate any violation of Dinah. For example, Johann S. Vater entitled his chapter simply "Jacob's Events at Shechem and his move to Bethel."[17] Heinrich

---

[13] Carl Friedrich Keil and Franz Delitzsch, eds., *The Pentateuch*, Biblical Commentary on the Old Testament, vol. 1, trans. James Martin (Grand Rapids, MI: Eerdmans, 1949), 311. For the original German see Carl Friedrich Keil, *Genesis und Exodus*, vol. 1, Biblischer Commentar über die Bücher Mose's, eds. C. F. Keil and F. Delitzsch (Leipzig: Dörffling & Franke, 1861), 224: "Cap XXXIV: Schändung der Dina und Rache Simeon's und Levi's."

[14] Peter von Bohlen, *Die Genesis historisch-kritisch erläutert* (Königsberg: Gebrüder Bornträger, 1835), 324: "Schwächung der Dina und Blutbad an Sichem."

[15] August Dillmann, *Die Genesis*, für die 3. Auflage nach Dr. August Knobel, Kurzgefasstes exegetisches Handbuch zum Alten Testament, Eilfte Lieferung, 3. verbesserte Auflage (Leipzig: S. Hirzel, 1875), 383: "Jacob bei Sikhem und die Entehrung der Dina."

[16] Hermann L. Strack, *Die Bücher Genesis, Exodus, Leviticus und Numeri*, Kurzgefasster Kommentar zu den heiligen Schriften Alten und Neuen Testamentes sowie zu den Apokryphen, A. AT. 1. Abt., eds. H. Strack & Otto Zöckler (Munich: C. H. Beck, 1894), 109: "Jakob in Sikhem. Simeon und Levi rächen die Entehrung der Dina."

[17] Johann Severin Vater, *Commentar über den Pentateuch, mit Einleitung zu den einzelnen Abschnitten, der Eingeschalteten Uebersetzung von Dr. Alexander Geddes's Merkwürdigeren Critischen und exegetischen Anmerkungen und einer Abhandlung über Moses und die Verfasser des Pentateuchs*, 3 vols., Erster Theil (Halle: Waisenhaus Buchhandlung, 1802), 279: "Begebenheiten Jacobs in der Gegend von Sichem, und sein Zug nach Bethel."

Holzinger used the ambiguous title "Complications with Shechem because of Dinah."[18] Gottfried Hoberg focused only on Jacob: "Jacob's Stay in Shechem: Chapter 34."[19] Stressing the fraternal revenge, Franz Delitzsch chose the title "Simeon's and Levi's Outrage at the Shechemites: 33:18-34."[20] Similarly, Michael Baumgarten opted for "Simeon's and Levi's Revenge against the Shechemites."[21] Lange was satisfied with listing topics: "Jacob's Settlement at Shechem; At Succoth; Dinah; Simeon and Levi; The first manifestation of Jewish fanaticism; Jacob's rebuking and removal to Bethel (33:17-35:15)."[22] Each of these titles reflected the perspective of the interpreter. Ignoring or minimizing Dinah's situation, they concentrated on Shechem, Jacob, or the brothers.

What the titles suggested, the interpretations confirmed. Several of them acknowledged the rape only to shift the focus to other topics. For Dillmann the fraternal response became the dominant issue. He explained that v. 2b referred to abduction and "rape" but had to be connected to v. 26 and to "all statements about the anger and malice of Dinah's brothers in 5. 7. 13. 31."[23] Dillmann at least acknowledged the rape as the standpoint from which to discuss the fraternal response. Friedrich W. J. Schröder stressed the aristocratic and privileged position of Shechem. Though Schröder used the word "rapist," he also simultaneously characterized him as the most respected son of the tribal sovereign Hamor.[24] Having called Shechem both rapist and aris-

---

[18] Holzinger, *Genesis*, 213: "Die Verwicklungen mit Sichem wegen der Dina."

[19] Hoberg, *Genesis*, 291: "Jakobs Aufenthalt bei Sichem. Kap. 34."

[20] Franz Delitzsch, *Die Genesis* (Leipzig: Dörffling & Franke, 1852), 339: "Simeons und Levi's Frevelthat an den Sichemiten XXXIII, 18. bis c. XXXIV." See also the title of the later edition of his *Neuer Commentar*, 1887, 411: "Der Aufenthalt in Sichem und Simeons und Levi's Rache wegen Dina's Entehrung XXXIII,18-c.XXXIV" (The Stay at Shechem and Simeon's and Levi's Revenge because of Dinah's Dishonoring).

[21] Michael Baumgarten, *Theologischer Commentar zum Pentateuch* (Kiel: Universitäts-Buchhandlung, 1843), 291: "Simeons und Levis Rache an den Sichemiten."

[22] Lange, Genesis or the First *Book of Moses*, 557.

[23] Dillmann, *Genesis*, 1882, 349: "alle die Aussagen über die Entrüstung und Tücke der Brüder der Dinah 5.7.13.31."

[24] Friedrich W. J. Schröder, *Das erste Buch Mose*, Das Alte Testament nach Dr. Martin Luther: Mit Einleitungen, berichtiger Uebersetzung und erklärenden Anmerkungen: Für Freunde des göttlichen Wortes, mit besonderer Rücksicht auf Lehrer in Kirchen und Schulen (Berlin: Justus Albert Wohlgemuth, 1846), 530: "Nothzüchtiger."

tocrat, Schröder ignored the meaning of the rape for Dinah. Hoberg
equated the rape with seduction. "Dinah was raped by Shechem, the
son of Hamor (vs. 1-2). Shechem and his father make preparations for
marriage . . . but Jacob's sons (Simeon and Levi) killed the seducer
. . . ."[25] For Hoberg the marriage preparations recast the rape as
seduction. Dinah is "the one who was seduced."[26] Hermann Gunkel
applied yet another strategy by acknowledging that a rape occurred in
Genesis 34, but only in one source.[27] By relegating the rape to the late
Priestly source, Gunkel even ignored the issue.

Some commentaries marginalized the phenomenon of rape by blaming Dinah for what happened. Baumgarten stated, "It is Dinah's punishable curiosity that she goes out to see the daughters of the land
because the daughters of Israel have nothing do with the daughters of
Canaan."[28] The interpretation then continued to discuss other topics.
Schröder made the point even more strongly when he argued that it
was wrong for Dinah "to visit them; a familiarity which is hardly appropriate for a daughter of Israel to do with the daughters of Canaan
(2 Cor. 6:17). Therefore, the punishment followed soon."[29] He supported his view with a reference to the New Testament and to his
understanding of nature:

> Dinah wird gewaltsam geschändet, weil sie, des Vaters Haus verlassend, freier
> herumstreift, als sie sollte. Sie hätte daheim bleiben sollen, wie der Apostel
> befiehlt (Tit. 2,5) und die Natur empfiehlt, denn auch die Jungfrauen, gleich
> den Ehefrauen, sollen Hüterinnen des Hauses sein.[30]

> Dinah is dishonored violently because she roams about more freely than she
> should, leaving the father's house. She should have stayed at home, as the

---

[25] Hoberg, *Genesis*, 291: "Dina wurde von Sichem, dem Sohne Hemors,
vergewaltigt (V. 1-2). Sichem wie sein Vater trafen Veranstaltungen, eine legitime
Ehe herbeizuführen . . . aber Jakobs Söhne (Simeon und Levi) ermordeten den
Verführer . . . ."
[26] Ibid., 292: "die Verführte."
[27] Hermann Gunkel, *Die Genesis*, Reihe Göttinger Handkommentar zum Alten
Testament, 1. verbesserte Auflage (Göttingen: Vandenhoeck & Rupprecht, 1901),
338.
[28] Baumgarten, *Genesis*, 292: "Es ist eine sträfliche Neugierde der Dina, daß sie
ausgeht die Töchter des Landes zu besehen, denn die Töchter Israels haben mit den
Töchtern Canaans Nichts zu schaffen."
[29] Schröder, *Erste Buch Moses*, 530: "sie zu besuchen; eine Vertraulichkeit, wie
sie der Tochter Israels mit den Töchtern Canaans schwerlich ziemt (2 Cor. 6, 17),
daher auch die Strafe nicht ausbleibt."
[30] Ibid.

apostle orders (Tit. 2:5) and nature recommends, because virgins, like wives, should be keepers of the house.

By blaming Dinah, Schröder marginalized the rape.

Other scholars followed suit. O. Naumann argued that Dinah was raped because she had inherited the wanton ways of her mother: "Shechem . . . dishonors Dinah, presumably not without her guilt, because the daughter inherited Lea's carnality."[31] Heinrich W. J. Thiersch presented another reason for Dinah's guilt; she did not receive her parents' permission and blessing before she left. He stated: "She missed what in such a situation youth needs as protection. Before she left, something was already wrong in her heart. Only this explains the fact that her trip ended in such a complete disaster."[32] Thiersch believed that "she put herself into danger and she perished in it" because of her "female curiosity and pertness." Dinah had a wrong attitude, and thus she invited the rape. As "there was no apology for Dinah," Thiersch moralized about her "miserable ending."[33]

Lange also blamed Dinah for the rape. For the most part his commentary on Genesis 34 used the terms "rape" and "seduction" indiscriminately. This confusion resulted from the belief that "some measure of consent on the part of Dinah is altogether probable."[34] Although at one point Lange acknowledged the word "seduction" as an "inadequate expression,"[35] he continued, "Dinah's history [is] a warning history for the daughters of Israel, and a foundation of the Old Testament's limitation of the freedom of the female sex."[36] Although Dinah's fate should serve as a cautionary tale to all women, Lange did not warn all rapists. "Seduction" remained the problem of Dinah alone and allowed Lange to ignore the implications of the rape.

---

[31] O. Naumann, *Das Erste Buch der Bibel nach seiner innteren Einheit und Echtheit* (Gütersloh: C. Bertelsmann, 1890), 217: "So hat Sichem . . . Dinah geschändet, wohl nicht ohne ihre Schuld, da der Lea Fleischeslust der Tochter Erbe wurde."

[32] Heinrich W. J. Thiersch, *Die Genesis nach ihrer moralischen und prophetischen Bedeutung* (Basel: Felix Schneider, 1870), 307: "Sie versäumte das, was in solchen Lagen der Jugend als Schutz notwendig ist. Es war bereits ehe sie ausging etwas in ihrem Herzen nicht richtig. Nur so war es möglich, daß es bei diesem Ausgang zu einem so tiefen Fall mit ihr kam."

[33] Ibid., 306, 307, 308.

[34] Lange, *Genesis*, 1884, 560.

[35] Ibid., 560.

[36] Ibid., 563f.

In the commentaries surveyed different emphases deflected attention from the rape. Some scholars, such as Bachmann, Baumgarten, Kurtz, and Strack, referred neither to rape nor to seduction, simply disregarding the incident. Some did not use the term "rape" in their titles, although their interpretations acknowledged it. The acknowledgment minimized or erased the significance of the event. Some, such as Gunkel and Holzinger,[37] referred to the rape only as a basis for discussing other topics. Others, such as Tuch, Thiersch, and Keil,[38] did not use the term "rape" but preferred the term "seduction." Some, such as Lange, blamed Dinah. As a group they all marginalized the rape.

Condemnation and Subtle Identification

Condemning Comments

Except for Dinah, the main characters in Genesis 34 are male: her brothers, Shechem, and the fathers Jacob and Hamor. Commentators evaluated their actions. Those who judged the brothers condemned them for their violent revenge. For instance, Dillmann evaluated the brothers as "malicious" both for holding tribal honor above all else and for using circumcision as a trick to kill the Shechemites.[39] He considered the fraternal reaction to Dinah's rape as "tribal pride" and dismissed it as narrowness. Delitzsch deemed the brothers deceitful. Despite their extraordinary "energetic moral purity" and the lacking judgment from the narrator, Delitzsch believed that the fraternal misuse of the "sacred sign of the covenant to so base a means of malice" was sinful.[40] The whole story showed "the disgrace of the promised generation not hiding how Simeon and Levi abused the sacred sign of covenant as deception for their private execrable revenge."[41] His colleague Keil lamented that although "their indignation was justifiable

---

[37] H. Holzinger, *Genesis* (Freiburg: Mohr, 1898), especially p. 216.

[38] Friedrich Tuch, *Commentar über die Genesis*, 2. Auflage besorgt von A. Arnold, nebst einem Nachwort von A. Merz (Halle: Buchhandlung des Waisenhauses, 1871), 406: "Dina, die Tochter Leas, wird von Sichem, einem hevitischen Stammesfürsten verführt;" Thiersch, *Genesis*, 305; Keil, *Pentateuch*, 311, 312.

[39] Dillmann, *Genesis*, 1875, 373, 375; see also Holzinger, *Genesis*, 213, 216.

[40] Delitzsch, *New Commentary*, 1889, 225f.

[41] Delitzsch, *Genesis*, 1852, 341: "Die ganze Geschichte . . . zeigt uns, die Schande des Verheissungsgeschlechts nicht bemäntelnd, wie das heilige Bundeszeichen von Simeon und Levi zum Trugmittel einer fluchwürdigen Privatrache gemissbraucht ward."

enough, the way the brothers rejected the Shechemites was wrong." They deceived the Shechemites, abused the covenant sign of circumcision, and extended the revenge to the whole city. Moreover, Jacob's "crafty character" degenerated "into malicious cunning in Simeon and Levi, and jealousy for the exalted vocation of their family, into actual sin." The last words of Jacob in Genesis 49:5-7 provided "sufficient proof that the wickedness of their conduct was also an object of deep abhorrence."[42] In other words these commentators rejected any sympathetic consideration of the brothers whom they characterized as sinful, abhorrent, and wicked.

Continuing the condemnation, Naumann judged the fraternal revenge "as a remarkable example of religious intolerance,"[43] and the "means of fighting" as immoral and full of "falsehood and deceit."[44] Christian C. Bunsen was disgusted by "the horrible and degrading revenge of the brothers."[45] Schröder deemed the brothers cruel, greedy, crude, and carnal characters. They were "men of blood" and "robbers who broke the covenant."[46] He believed that Jacob's judgment in Genesis 49:5-7 gave appropriate punishment to his sons Simeon and Levi:

> Darum ist diese Unthat hier, bei welcher Simeon und Levi nur ihre Privatrache im Auge hatten, anstatt die Rache dem Herrn zu überlassen, so unnachsichtlich geahndet worden.[47]

> That is why their misdeed, in which Simeon and Levi focused only on their private revenge instead of leaving revenge to the Lord, is so severely punished.

Lange's interpretation also disclosed his hostile evaluation of the brothers by calling their act "fanatical." He believed that "their resort to subtle and fanatical conduct merits only a hearty condemnation."[48]

---

[42] Keil, *Biblical Commentary*, 315.

[43] Bohlen, *Genesis*, 326.

[44] Naumann, *Erste Buch Moses*, 218.

[45] Christian C. Bunsen, *Die Bibel oder die Schriften des Alten und Neuen Bundes nach den überlieferten Grundtexten übersetzt und für die Gemeinde erklärt: Vollständiges Bibelwerk für die Gemeinde, in 3 Abtheilungen*, Erste Abtheilung: *Die Bibel: Uebersetzung und Erklärung*: Erster Theil: *Das Gesetz* (Leipzig: F. A. Brockhaus, 1858), 72: "die entsetzliche und unmenschliche Rache der Brüder."

[46] Schröder, *Erste Buch Mose*, 532.

[47] Ibid., 533.

[48] Lange, *Genesis*, 1884, 561. See the section "Orientalism instead of Rape" for the problem of anti-Judaism in these commentaries.

For him the story is "the birthplace of Jewish fanaticism."[49] He viewed "this narrative as the history of the origin and first original form of Jewish and Christian fanaticism," and presented examples from the Christian tradition for "this Shechemite carnage of blind and Jewish fanaticism." Here the brothers represented "Jewish fanaticism," whereas Jacob "justly declares his condemnation of the iniquity of the brothers not only at once but also upon his deathbed (ch. XLIX)."[50]

According to Lange, Jacob rightly condemned his sons because they were "full of cunning, falsehood, and cruelty." Lange appreciated the fact that the narrator did not hesitate to bring "into prominence whatever traits of excellence there were in the characters of Shechem and Hamor."[51] This complex interpretation related the fraternal "guilt of fanaticism" to Jacob's task in Genesis 35 where the father needed to purify his house of the fanaticism of his sons:

> As Jacob intends holding a feast of praise and thanksgiving at Bethel, he enjoins upon his household first a feast of purification . . . . But it is to be observed here that Jacob is first sealed after having purified his faith from any share in the guilt of fanaticism.[52]

Lange sympathized with Jacob, Shechem, and Shechem's father Hamor. The brothers, however, exemplified fanaticism which "either discredit[s] Christianity in the moral estimate of the world, and imperil[s] its very existence by its unreasonable zeal, or . . . expose[s] it to the most severe persecutions."[53] Clearly, the fraternal revenge received detailed attention, but Lange never related it directly to the rape.

From this overwhelming condemnation one can infer that the commentators sided with the rapist. Delitzsch commented:

> Da sieht sie Schechem, der Sohn des Landesfürsten, bringt sie zu Falle und vermag sich von ihr, der Liebgewonnenen, nicht mehr zu trennen. . . . Der junge Fürst beeilte sich aus Liebe zu Dina, diese Bedingung [der Brüder] zu erfüllen.[54]

> Shechem, the son of the ruler, sees her, causes her to fall, and is no longer able to leave from the loved one . . . . Because of his love toward Dinah, the young prince hurried to fulfill the conditions [of the brothers].

---

[49] Ibid., 563.
[50] Ibid., 564
[51] Ibid.
[52] Ibid., 565.
[53] Ibid., 564.
[54] Delitzsch, *Genesis*, 1852, 340.

In this interpretation the rapist became the lover of Dinah. Dillmann also emphasized Shechem's love. He wrote that Shechem "spoke to her heart and sought to comfort her with his love and with the future about the past events."[55] Gunkel repeatedly mentioned Shechem's love: "Because he loves Dinah, he soothes her, and promises to marry her;" and "because he loves her, he asks his father to court for her;" and "the enarmored Shechem accepts immediately the conditions."[56] Lange not only stated that "Shechem . . . passionately loves and would marry the dishonored maiden and is ready to pay any sum as an atonement,"[57] but he also imagined that Dinah consented: "Judging from Dinah's levity, it [the rape] was not without her consent."[58] Imagining that Dinah consented and that Shechem was in love, the brothers became truly despicable. Commentators condemned them.

Mixed Comments

A few scholars departed from the overwhelming condemnation of the brothers to suggest a positive aspect to their deeds. Baumgarten assigned to the brothers a "noble indignation."[59] Yet in the end he turned to the familiar view that "this dispersion of Simeon and Levi is the appropriate punishment for their union which was against the spirit of Israel . . . against the will of Yahwe."[60] Referring to Genesis 49:5-7, Baumgarten argued that Jacob spoke against his sons "with the spirit of the holy God," punishing them for "anger and revenge."[61]

In juggling the fraternal response and the rape, Thiersch made an intriguing link between the brothers' behavior and his own contemporaries:

> Was sollen wir sagen von der schrecklichen Rache, welche diese Männer für die geraubte Ehre und Unschuld ihrer Schwester genommen haben? In einer

---

[55] Dillmann, *Genesis*, 1875, 386: "[Er] redete ihr zu Herzen, suchte sie mit seiner Liebe und mit der Zukunft über das Geschehene zu beruhigen." See his other comments on p. 386: "An die Gewaltthat schliesst sich Liebe zu der Geschwächten;" on p. 388: "Weil Sikhem die Dinah so lieb hatte, zögerte er nicht, die Beschneidung anzunehmen."

[56] Gunkel, *Genesis*, 336. See also Schröder, *Genesis*, 531.

[57] Lange, *Genesis*, 564.

[58] Ibid., 567.

[59] Baumgarten, *Commentar*, 292: "edler Unwille."

[60] Ibid., 369: "Diese Zerstreuung Simeons and Levis ist die angemessene Strafe für ihre Verbindung, welche wider den Geist Israels war . . . wider den Willen Jehovas."

[61] Ibid., 368: "Zornmuth und Rachegeist."

Hinsicht muß man sie loben, und ihr Eifer hat etwas ruhmwürdiges, wenn
man ihn mit der entsetzlichen Stumpfheit und Gefühlslosigkeit vergleicht, womit
in unserer Zeit und Umgebung manche, die doch den Christennamen tragen,
solche schändliche Thaten mit ansehen und an sich vorübergehen lassen, als
wäre nichts besonderes vorgefallen.[62]

What should we say about the dreadful revenge which these men took for the
stolen honor and innocence of their sister? In one aspect one has to praise
them, and their zeal is praiseworthy if one compares it to the terrible dullness
and unfeelingness with which in our time and place some who carry the
name of Christ watch such scandalous deeds and let them go as if nothing
special had happened.

Although Thiersch did not explicitly mention the rape, he complained
that his contemporaries ignored "such scandalous deeds." By contrast, then, the reaction of the brothers appeared almost commendable.

Muted Comments

The commentaries by Strack, Gunkel, and Tuch took a muted stance
toward the fraternal response. Strack wrote that "the conduct of Simeon
and Levi is not explicitly judged by the narrator."[63] Interested primarily
in grammatical, stylistic, and historical analyses, Strack refrained from
evaluative remarks, although he admitted that "very often the Old
Testament which becomes holy through its neutrality—particularly in
its older parts—leaves it to the reader to draw the lesson from the
narrative."[64] And so he welcomed Jacob's cursing of his sons in Genesis 49:5-7, perhaps an indication of his negative opinion about the
sons:

Die Handlungsweise Simeons und Levis wird seitens der biblischen
Geschichtsdarstellung nicht ausdrücklich beurteilt . . . . Gar oft überläßt die
auch durch ihre Unparteilichkeit als heilig sich erweisende heilige Schrift Alten
Testaments, zumal in ihren älteren Teilen, es dem Leser, aus der Geschichte
die Lehre selbst zu ziehen. Gleichsam aber damit kein Vorwitziger es wage
auf Grund solcher schlichten Aneinanderreihung historischer Überlieferungen
eine Anklage wegen Mangels an sittlichem Ernste auszusprechen, hat sie an
andren Stellen in ganz andrem Zusammenhange ernste Urteile über manches
Ereignis aufbewahrt. So über Simeon und Levi in Jakobs letzten Worten 49,
5-7.[65]

---

[62] Thiersch, *Genesis*, 309.
[63] Strack, *Genesis*, 111.
[64] Ibid.
[65] Ibid.

The activity of Simeon and Levi is not explicitly judged in the biblical narrative . . . Showing its holiness through its impartiality, often Holy Scripture
leaves it to the reader to draw the conclusion for himself, especially in its
older parts. So that no presumptuous reader dares to formulate an accusation
because of a lack of moral seriousness, scripture also preserved serious judgment about many events in other contexts. For example, this is the case
concerning Simeon and Levi in Jacob's final words in 49:5-7.

Gunkel also refrained from giving a clear judgment, although he
referred to the "enamored Shechem"[66] in contrast to "the most vehe-
mently infuriated blood brothers."[67] This characterization of the rapist
and the brothers seems to beg the question why the brothers were so
infuriated, if Shechem was truly in love. Indirectly, Gunkel seems therefore to side with the rapist Shechem. Another commentator, Tuch, did
not judge the brothers, Jacob, or Shechem. He stated that "by no
means does the present narrative criticize Simeon and Levi who punish a crime that deserves the death penalty from the Hebrew perspective."[68] But Tuch also argued that Jacob encountered a challenge which
"attaches a stain to his tribal honor."[69] This phrase hints at an opinion
about the brothers, although the commentary deals primarily with
historical critical questions.

In condemning the severe response of the brothers to the "assault"
by Shechem, some biblical commentators of the nineteenth century
minimized Dinah's experience. They considered the fraternal deeds to
be out of proportion to the crime, and thus they identified subtly with
the rapist.

Rape and Love
The commentaries defined rape in a variety of ways. One prominent
way characterized what Shechem did as an expression of love and
thus implied that "love" erased rape and its significance. Delitzsch
believed that "the young seducer only loved her whom he had seduced
the more, soothed her with pleasant prospects of the future, and actually entreated his father to take him the damsel for a wife. . . . Shechem
really loved Dinah."[70] Delitzsch imagined that Shechem hurried to ful-

---

[66] Gunkel, *Die Genesis*, 336, 339.

[67] Ibid., 339.

[68] Tuch, *Genesis*, 408: "Die vorliegende Erzählung will im mindesten keinen
Tadel gegen Simeon und Levi aussprechen, welche hier ein vom Standpuncte des
Hebräerthums todeswürdiges Verbrechen nach Verdienst züchtigen."

[69] Ibid., 406: "der Ehre seines Stammes einen Makel anheftet."

[70] Delitzsch, *New Commentary*, 1894, 219, 222.

fill the fraternal demand for circumcision because he loved Dinah so much.[71] Dillmann saw no contradiction when he stated that "after the violent act follows love for the weakened," that is, for Dinah.[72] His colleague Keil argued that "Shechem . . . sought to comfort her by the promise of a happy marriage."[73] Hoberg considered the love of Shechem an "awakening" one, leading him to desire "legitimate marriage."[74]

Other scholars also adopted this view about Shechem. Lange believed that the expression "his soul clave unto Dinah" disclosed that Shechem's act was "not an act of pure, simple lust, which usually regards its subject with hatred . . . ."[75] This statement exemplified Lange's belief that the definition of rape depended on what the rapist felt. For Lange, only "pure, simple lust" turned a man into a rapist. Love and the promise of an "honorable" marriage erased the sexual assault. Accepting the genuineness of Shechem's love, Lange absolved Shechem from the rape. Gunkel also believed that Shechem "started loving Dinah, soothed her, and promised to marry her."[76] So deeply in love with Dinah, Shechem immediately accepted the fraternal demands.[77] Referring to Shechem's speech in vv. 11-12, Gunkel said, "A listener likes to hear that such a noble Canaanite takes such pains over an Israelite girl."[78]

No criticism of the rapist emerged from these scholarly interpretations—only admiration and appreciation of Shechem's love. In other words scholars mitigated the rape by dwelling on love. They accepted that rape could become love. Love could incorporate rape. In redefining the rape commentators sympathized with the rapist.

Rape versus Maturity

The age of Dinah was a topic of interest to biblical scholars, though Genesis 34 is silent on the subject. A few scholars pointed out that the narrated chronology is unclear, making the calculation of Dinah's age difficult. Holzinger stated that "Dinah's marriageability made no chro-

---

[71] Delitzsch, *Genesis*, 1852, 340.

[72] Dillmann, *Genesis*, 1875, 386.

[73] Keil, *Pentateuch*, 312.

[74] Hoberg, *Genesis*, 291, 292.

[75] Lange, *Genesis*, 1884, 560.

[76] Gunkel, *Genesis*, 1901, 336: "Er [gewinnt] Dina lieb, beruhigt sie und verspricht ihr die Heirat."

[77] Ibid.

[78] Ibid., 340.

nological sense in the Jahwist and Elohist sources."[79] Bohlen pointed
out the lack of textual unclarity concerning Dinah's age. She could
have been just six or seven years old "because Jacob married Leah
only after seven years of work, Dinah is the seventh child of Leah, and
he stayed only twenty years with Laban."[80] Both commentators dismissed the possibility of establishing Dinah's age but considered the
question valid.

Other scholars were more optimistic about the possibility. Dillmann
suggested that she was twelve years old.[81] Calculating Benjamin's date
of birth in relation to Joseph's age, Baumgarten rejected Bohlen's
proposal of six to seven years. His Dinah was thirteen years old because "we do not know for how long Jacob stayed at Succoth . . . ."[82]
Schröder believed that Dinah was sixteen years old because "the event
occurs ten years after Jacob's return from Mesopotamia."[83] At first
Delitzsch agreed,[84] but he later reduced Dinah's age from sixteen to
fourteen years.[85] Acknowledging the diversity of opinions, Keil also
calculated Dinah's age. He argued that she had been five years old
when Jacob had left Mesopotamia eight to ten years earlier, so that
she must have been sixteen years old at the time of the rape.[86] Lange
embraced the spectrum by asserting that Dinah was between twelve
and sixteen years old, most probably fourteen or fifteen.[87] Gunkel simply wrote, "Dinah is a grown-up girl."[88]

As we will see in the next chapter on forensic medicine, this ab-
sorption with the age of Dinah is reminiscent of debates about establishing the maturity of a young woman. Considering the possibility
that a girl might look older than her chronological age, forensic scholars were ready to protect the alleged rapist. Since German laws pun-

---

[79] Holzinger, *Genesis*, 215: "Wie die Mannbarkeit der Dina chronologisch sich in
JE einfügt, muss auf sich beruhen."

[80] Bohlen, *Genesis*, 327: "insofern der Patriarch die Lea erst nach den sieben
Dinstjahren erhielt, Dina das siebente Kind der Lea ist, und er nur 20 Jahre bey
Laban geblieben war."

[81] Dillmann, *Genesis*, 1875, 386.

[82] Baumgarten, *Commentar*, 291.

[83] Schröder, *Erste Buch Mose*, 529: "Die Begebenheit überhaupt fiel 10 Jahre
nach Jakobs Rückkehr aus Mesopotamien vor."

[84] Delitzsch, *Genesis*, 1852, 340.

[85] Delitzsch, *New Commentary*, II, 1889, 219.

[86] Keil, *Pentateuch*, 311f.

[87] Lange, *Genesis*, 1884, 560.

[88] Gunkel, *Genesis*, 340: "Dina ist ein erwachsenes Mädchen."

ished any sexual contact with a girl below the age of fourteen years—
sometimes below twelve years—forensic scholars were obliged to make
a judgment about the age of a raped girl, based on her physical appearance. Although biblical scholars did not refer explicitly to the law
codes, their speculations relate them to the forensic discussions about
maturity. Furthermore their judgment often reflected those of forensic
authorities. As age can mitigate rape, so Dinah's maturity could excuse Shechem from charges of rape.

Orientalism instead of Rape

Several commentaries relied on the concept of Orientalism[89] to explain behavior in Genesis 34 which they found alien to their own
culture. Orientalism was "a way of coming to terms with the Orient
that is based on the Orient's special place in European Western experience."[90] Several scholars relied on information from travellers to the
Middle East to illuminate the fraternal response as an "oriental" phenomenon.[91] So Bohlen explained that the killing of the Shechemites
corresponded to "customs of the East . . . because the brother defends
the innocence of his sister by all means and revenges her dishonor
more than he does for his wife, whom he can expel."[92] Schröder referred to "southern Asia, where the brother is more offended by the
dishonoring of his sister than the man is by his wife's unfaithfulness
because—so Arabian men say—a man can divorce his wife and then
she is no longer his. A sister and daughter, however, remain sister and
daughter forever."[93] Lange stated that "seduction is punished with death

---

[89] For the classic treatment of Orientalism see Edward W. Said, *Orientalism* (New
York: Vintage, 1979).

[90] Ibid., 1.

[91] See, for example, references in Dillmann, *Genesis*, 1892, 374; Keil, *Genesis*,
1861, 227, to the travel guide book by John L. Burckhardt, *Reisen in Syrien,
Palästina und der Gegend des Berges Sinai*, trans. by W. Gesenius (Weimar, 1823-
24).

[92] Bohlen, *Genesis*, 326: "den Sitten des Morgenlandes . . . denn der Bruder hat
die Unschuld seiner Schwester auf alle Weise zu vertheidigen, und eine an ihr
begangene Schmach mehr zu rächen, als wäre sie seinem Weibe, welches er verstossen
kann, widerfahren."

[93] Schröder, *Erste Buch Mose*, 531: "[Man glaubt] im südlichen Asien, daß der
Bruder durch die Entehrung seiner Schwester mehr beleidigt werde, als der Mann
durch die Untreue seiner Frau, denn, sagen noch jetzt die Araber, der Mann kann
sich von seiner Frau scheiden, und dann ist sie nicht mehr sein; Schwester und
Tochter aber bleibt ewig Schwester und Tochter." See also Bunsen, *Bibel*, 72;
Dillmann, *Genesis*, 1875, 389.

among the Arabians, and the brothers of the seduced are generally active in inflicting it."[94] The idea of "the wild Eastern vindictiveness"[95] gave these commentators an opportunity to interpret the brothers as the "Other." Not reflecting on the significance of the rape or the rapist, they explained the fraternal response as a custom of the "Orient."

Commentators not only qualified the behavior of the brothers by calling them "Orientals." They also argued that Dinah's maturity and Shechem's nature were of "Oriental" origin. Referring to Dinah, Schröder believed that "in the Orient female maturity can start at twelve, sometimes even ten years."[96] Keil and Baumgarten agreed that maturity "is often the case in the East at the age of twelve, and sometimes earlier."[97] Shechem's heritage was reflected in the "Oriental despot" Abimelech and also in David. Both were driven by the "instinct of nature" and were stimulated by "sexual change, rarity, or the strangeness of the case."[98] The concept called Orientalism was used to excuse rape.

A connection between Orientalism and anti-Judaism became obvious in Lange's commentary. He characterized the actions of Simeon and Levi as "the wild Eastern vindictiveness" and "the birthplace of Jewish fanaticism."[99] According to Lange, "Israelitish pride" caused the revenge.[100] Lange symbolized the revenge of the brothers with the phrase "the smoke of zealousness." He then appropriated Jacob for Christian purposes, characterizing Jacob's response with the phrase "the pure flame of faith." Lange explained:

> In all actual individual cases, it is a question whether the flame overcomes the smoke, or the smoke the flame. In the life of Christ, the Old Testament covenant faithfulness and truth burns pure and bright, entirely free from smoke; in the history of old Judaism, on the contrary, a dangerous mixture of fire and

---

[94] Lange, *Genesis*, 1884, 561. For an appraisal of the brothers' prevention of "mixed heathenish marriages" see Naumann, *Genesis*, 218.

[95] Ibid., 567.

[96] Schröder, *Erste Buch Mose*, 530: "daß die Mannbarkeit des weiblichen Geschlechts im Morgenland schon mit 12 ja mit 10 Jahren eintreten kann . . . ."

[97] Keil, *Genesis*, 224: "da im Morgenlande die geschlechtliche Reife schon mit dem 12. Jahre, auch wohl noch früher einzutreten pflegt;" Baumgarten, *Pentateuch*, 291f.

[98] Schröder, *Erste Buch Mose*, 384: "der Wechsel, oft die Seltenheit, ja die Absonderlichkeit eines Falles."

[99] Lange, *Genesis*, 1884, 567, 561.

[100] Ibid., 561.

smoke steams over the land. And so in the development of individual believers we see how some purify themselves to the purest Christian humanity,
while others, ever sinking more and more into the pride, cunning, and un-
charitableness and injustice of fanaticism are completely ruined.[101]

Like many of his colleagues Lange participated in the long Christian
tradition of elevating Christianity by denigrating Judaism. The condemnation of the brothers was one way to combine prejudices about
both Arabs ("Orientals") and Jews. In a larger way such discussions
divert attention from the subject of rape.

* * * * * * * * *

An investigation of Genesis 34 in commentaries written by Christians in nineteenth-century Germany has isolated five major ideas about
rape.

1) Scholars marginalized rape in the chapter titles and expositions.
2) They condemned the brothers and identified with Shechem.
3) They homogenized rape with love.
4) They emphasized Dinah's maturity to belittle the rape.
5) They introduced the concept of Orientalism to divert from the
   issue of rape.

One might think that the biblical-theological discourse accounts for
these peculiar notions on rape. However, the next chapter will provide evidence that the so-called scientific field did not fare much better. An example for the cultural context of nineteenth-century Germany, forensic medical textbooks contain views comparable to the
commentaries.

---

[101] Ibid., 564.

Chapter 4

Retrospecting Rape (Part Two): Forensic Medical Textbooks of Nineteenth-Century Germany

Ideas about rape in forensic medical textbooks of nineteenth-century Germany emerged from a broader cultural context—a context that includes biblical commentaries of the time. As a result, the views of such commentaries cannot be simply dismissed for their religious-theological origin.

Two reasons led to the choice of the forensic medical textbooks. One reason refers to the discipline of medicine. The philosopher Michel Foucault argued that the modern discourse on sexuality developed early in the nineteenth century when institutions of social control medicalized sex.[1] The discourse on sexuality was historically specific and emerged within "a subtle network of discourses."[2] Forensic medicine participated in the process of describing and interpreting sexuality in scientific terms, and rape was one aspect of that discourse because medicine played such a crucial role in the development of the discourse on sexuality, forensic textbooks participated in "the expanding production of discourse on sex."[3] Forensic medicine represents, then, an adequate example for the general nineteenth-century discourse on rape.

The other reason refers to the genre of the "textbook" which represents a solid and accessible source for examining ideas on rape in the

------

[1] Michel Foucault, *The History of Sexuality*, vol. 1: *An Introduction*, transl. Robert Hurley (New York: Random House, 1978), 65, 117, 119.

[2] Ibid., 72.

[3] Ibid., 98.

nineteenth-century discipline of medicine. A large number of textbooks introduced students, teachers, and physicians to all the major topics of the discipline. They regularly contained a section on rape. In contrast to individual articles and essays, textbooks were central in the education of forensic medical professionals. Moreover, the selection of a particular genre provides a concise and coherent way to study forensic medical ideas on rape.[4]

A word of caution, however. The relationship of forensic medical textbooks and biblical commentaries promotes intertextual reading strategies but does not posit causal links. The analysis will not prove that biblical scholars literally interacted with forensic researchers or that they themselves had read the textbooks. Rather, the correlation provides a solid rationale for evaluating the ideas on rape. The connection between textbooks and commentaries is a cultural, not a causal, relationship. Another example from this cultural context might suggest conclusions different from those proposed here. However, as suggested by Foucault, forensic medical textbooks represent an excellent source for understanding ideas about rape in the commentaries because modern medical discourse developed during the nineteenth century.

Questions of Terminology

A modern definition of forensic medicine calls it "a science that deals with the relation and application of medical facts to legal problems."[5] The definition of the term "forensic medicine" is, however, not as simple as the dictionary makes it appear. Nineteenth-century forensic medicine used various terms such as "*Gerichtliche Physik*," "*Gerichtliche Arzneywissenschaft*," "*Gerichtliche Staats-Arzneywissenschaft*," "*Medicinische Polizeywissenschaft*," and "*Gerichtliche Medizin*." Forensic physicians were sometimes called "medical police" in the eighteenth century. Nineteenth-century German terminology identified the courtroom situation as the primary location and consequently used the term "*Gerichtliche Medizin*" (courtroom or

---

[4] For this last argument see Anke Meyer-Knees, *Verführung und sexuelle Gewalt: Untersuchung zum medizinischen und juristischen Diskurs im 18. Jahrhundert*, Probleme der Semiotik, Band 12 (Tübingen: Stauffenburg, 1992), 72.

[5] *Webster's Ninth New Collegiate Dictionary* (Springfield, MA: Merriam-Webster, 1991).

juridicial medicine). Influenced by the French "*médicine légale,*" the term "legal medicine" rather than "forensic medicine" gained popularity in the English-speaking world. Different linguistic settings yielded different terminology. Insisting on the authority of the founders of forensic medicine, the German scholar I. H. Schürmayer wrote in 1854:

> Die neueste Zeit hat, und mit Recht, wieder für die von Bohn zuerst gebrauchte Benennung "gerichtliche Medizin"—Medicine forensis—entschieden, so dass dieser Name zuversichtlich der herrschende bleiben dürfte.[6]

> Recent times have decided again, and rightly so, in favor of the earliest terminology (first used by Bohn) "courtroom medicine"—medicine forensis—so that this name will probably remain the dominant one.[7]

The statement illustrates the early effort to bring terminological coherence to the field but it also leads to the question how to translate the various titles used in the textbooks.

In 1975, William J. Curran suggested that the interdisciplinary character of forensic medicine caused the confusion of titles.[8] Pointing to historical developments, he attempted to clarify the terminology. The Latin "*forensis*" referred to the common meeting place of ancient Roman culture, where goods were exchanged, speeches were made, and legal affairs were settled. In English the word "forensic" referred to either public speaking and debating or legal and court affairs. Accordingly, forensic medicine is that part of medicine which is concerned with the presentation of medical data in courts. In 1977, Bernard J. Fiacarra came to a similar conclusion, arguing that the term "forensic medicine" characterized "the use of medical science to elucidate legal problems."[9] Likewise, Catherine Crawford explained in

---

[6] I. H. Schürmayer, *Lehrbuch der Gerichtlichen Medicin: Mit Berücksichtigung der neueren Gesetzgebungen des In- und Auslandes insbesondere des Verfahrens bei Schwurgerichten. Für Ärzte und Juristen,* mit einem Nachwort, 2. Auflage (Erlangen: Ferdinand Enke, 1854).

[7] All translations are mine unless indicated otherwise. The aim of these translations is not to render them into fluent English but to convey the flavor of the German. If the German is awkward, the English is awkward. For example, the awkward syntax and word choice of the quote on p. 67 results in an awkward translation.

[8] William J. Curran, "The Confusion of Titles in the Medicolegal Field: An Historical Analysis and a Proposal for Reform," *Medicine, Science and the Law* 15 (1975): 270-75. The following explanations rely on this article.

[9] Bernard J. Fiacarra, "History of Legal Medicine," *Legal Medicine Annual 1976* (1977): 3-4.

Encyclopedia of the History of Medicine that "it is now usual to reserve 'forensic medicine' for medicine relating to law courts and regulating bodies."[10] Hence, this study translates the various terms with "forensic medicine."

Historical Overview of German Forensic Medicine

Forensic medicine started with the *Constitutio criminalis Carolina (Peinliche Halsgerichtsordnung)*, or the Caroline Code, published and proclaimed by the German Emperor Charles V in 1533. Based on the *Constitutio Bambergensis* of 1507, the Caroline Code instructed courts to obtain expert medical testimony, though several articles dealt with issues that did not require such advice. Among these articles was paragraph 119 on rape:

> So jemand einer unverleumden Ehe-Frau, Wittben, oder Jungfrauen mit Gewalt oder wider ihren Willen ihre jungfräuliche oder fräuliche Ehre nehme, derselbige Uebelthäter hat das Leben verwürkt, und soll auf Beklagung der Benöthigten, in Ausführung der Missethat einem Räuber gleich, mit dem Schwerdte vom Leben zum Tode gerichtet werden. So sich aber einer solches obgemeldtes Mißhandels freventlicher und gewaltsamer Weise gegen einer unverleumdeten Frauen oder Jungfrauen unterstünde, und sich die Frau oder Jungfrau sein erwehrete, oder von solcher Beschwerniß sonst errettet würde, derselbige Uebelthäter soll auf Beklagung der Benöthigten in Ausführung der Mißhandlung, nach Gelegenheit und Gestalt der Personen und unterstandenen Missethat gestraft werden, und sollen darinnen Richter und Urtheiler Raths gebrauchen.[11]

> If someone takes the honor of an honorable wife or virgin with force or against her will, this wrongdoer has lost his life. Upon accusation by the forced female he is to be put to death with the sword, similar to a robber. If a male committed such an announced criminal and violent mistreatment, and if the woman or virgin resisted or in some other way was rescued from the hardship, this wrongdoer has to be punished according to opportunity and the

---

[10] Catherine Crawford, "Medicine and the Law," in *Encylopedia of the History of Medicine*, ed. W. F. Bynum and Roy Porter, vol. 2 (London: Routledge, 1993), 1620.

[11] The text is quoted in Johann Valentin Müller, *Entwurf der gerichtlichen Arzneywissenschaft nach juristischen und medicinischen Grundsätzen für Geistliche, Rechtsgelehrte und Aerzte*, Erster Band von den Materien, welche denen Ehegerichten zur Entscheidung vorgelegt werden (Frankfurt/Main: Andreäische Buchhandlung, 1796), 119.

appearance of the persons and the announced misdeed. Moreover, the advice of judges and evaluators should be used.

Although the Caroline Code did not consistently require medical testimony, as in the above paragraph, nevertheless it became the basis for the development of forensic medicine as an independent discipline.[12] The inconsistency still astounds scholars. Commenting on the lack of medical judgment in the paragraph on rape, Robert P. Brittain wrote: "It seems impossible that there was not such intervention."[13]

After the sixteenth century, forensic medicine matured in France, Italy, and especially Germany. The historian Erwin H. Ackerknecht speaks of a "German monopoly" after the seventeenth century,[14] a period in which German scholars such as Albert Michaelis and Johannes Bohn developed definitions and methods. In the eighteenth century scientists such as Joseph J. Plenck and Johann D. Metzger furthered the establishment of university chairs in forensic medicine and systematically taught students of medicine and law.[15] Nineteenth-century German forensic professors praised the German contribution to the discipline, perhaps because of their patriotic bias. Adolph Henke, the famous forensic scholar of the period, wrote:

> Seit der Mitte des sechzehnten Jahrhunderts bildete sich also die gerichtliche Arzneikunde allmälig. Im siebzehnten Jahrhundert blieb jedoch die Wissenschaft noch in ihrer Kindheit . . . . Im achzehnten Jahrhundert wurde die gerichtliche Medicin durch die Bemühungen einer Reihe der vorzüglichsten und

---

[12] Cf. Erwin H. Ackerknecht, "Legal Medicine in Transition (16th-18th Centuries)," *Ciba Symposia* 11, no. 7 (Winter 1950-1951) 1290-1298; Robert P. Brittain, "Origins of Legal Medicine: Constitution Criminalis Carolina," *Medicolegal Journal* 33 (1965): 124-27; Catherine Crawford, "Legalizing Medicine: Early Modern Legal Systems and the Growth of Medico-Legal Knowledge," in *Legal Medicine in History*, ed. Michael Clark and Catherine Crawford (Cambridge, UK: Cambridge University Press, 1994), 89-116; Crawford, "Medicine and the Law," 1619-1640; Ficarra, "History of Legal Medicine," 3-27; Jaroslav Nemec, *Highlights in Medicolegal Relations*, rev. and enlarged ed. (Bethesda, MD: U.S. Department of Health, Education and Welfare, 1976); Sydney Alfred Smith, "The History and Development of Legal Medicine," in *Legal Medicine*, ed. R. B. H. Gradwohl (St. Louis: Mosby, 1954), 1-19.

[13] Robert P. Brittain, "Origins of Legal Medicine: Constitutio Criminalis Carolina," *Medicolegal Journal* 33 (1965): 124.

[14] Ackerknecht, "Legal Medicine," 1296.

[15] Sydney Alfred Smith, "The History and Development of Legal Medicine," in *Legal Medicine*, 9f; Ficarra, "History of Legal Medicine," 7.

scharfsinnigsten Aerzte, vorzüglich deutscher Nation, allmälig immer mehr vervolkommnet.[16]

Since the middle of the sixteenth century forensic medicine was slowly developed. During the seventeenth century the science was in its childhood. . . . During the eighteenth century forensic medicine was more and more improved through the efforts of a number of excellent and intelligent physicians, among them many of German origin.

During the nineteenth century many university positions were created to teach and promote forensic medicine. Students were increasingly interested in the subject. A flood of textbooks was written and published. The systematic documentation about the observations of corpses and living bodies makes textbooks a rich source for many topics, and not only rape.[17]

Of the large number of textbooks produced in this century, three were especially significant. The first, published by Adolf C. H. Henke (1775-1843), became the standard textbook early in the century.[18] The first edition appeared in 1812. The thirteenth and last edition appeared posthumously in 1859. A professor at the University of Erlangen, Henke was a recognized expert in the field, even though Johann L. Casper, a former student, criticized him scathingly:

He had never performed one judicial dissection, never stepped across the threshold of any prison, never examined any woman said to have been de-

---

[16] Adolph C. H. Henke, *Lehrbuch der Gerichtlichen Medizin: Zum Behufe academischer Vorlesungen und zum Gebrauch für gerichtliche Ärzte und Rechtsgelehrte entworfen*, 13. Auflage mit Nachträgen von Carl Bergmann (Berlin: Ferdinand Dümmler, 1859), 12. See also Wolfgang Friedrich Wilhelm Klose, *System der gerichtlichen Physik* (Breslau: Johann Friedrich Korn, 1814), VIII: "Die gerichtliche Physik ist ihrer Entstehung und ihrer vorzüglichsten Ausbildung nach, als eine Deutsche Wissenschaft zu betrachten."

[17] See S. Placzek, "Geschichte der gerichtlichen Medizin," in *Handbuch der Geschichte der Medizin,* ed. Max Neuburger und Julius Page, vol. 3 (Jena: Gustav Fischer, 1905), 747. Many textbooks quote the various local German law codes which became unified in 1871 in the "Deutsche Strafgesetzbuch." See the Appendix for the local German laws valid until 1870 and for the unified German laws of 1871.

[18] Adolph C. H. Henke, *Lehrbuch der gerichtlichen Medicin: Zum Behufe academischer Vorlesungen und zum Gebrauch für gerichtliche Ärzte und Rechtsgelehrte entworfen* (Berlin: J. E. Hitzig, 1812). Editions: 1: 1812; 2: 1819; 3: 1821; 4: 1824; 5: 1827; 6: 1829; 7: 1832; 9: 1838; 10: 1841; 11: 1845; 12: 1851 (ed. by Bergmann); 13: 1859 (ed. by Bergmann).

flowered, never investigated the doubtful mental condition of even one criminal or of a single case of malignancy, or ever stood as an expert before any
court.[19]

Despite Casper's judgment, Henke's contribution remained undisputed.
As late as 1976 historian Jaroslav Nemec acknowledged Henke as
"the leading personality in legal medicine of his time."[20]

Johann Ludwig Casper (1796-1864) wrote the second major compendium, while a professor in Berlin. First published in 1858, this
book remained unsurpassed for decades; it went through nine editions and shortly after his death was translated into English.[21] Its characteristic feature was the integration of individual cases into general
discussions on forensic phenomena. In this way Casper modified the
general and universal statements, typical of other compendiums, by
describing specific cases.[22] Many subsequent textbooks followed his
lead.

The third book appeared in the latter part of the nineteenth century, written by Eduard von Hofmann (1837-1897), eight editions were
published during his lifetime, and two appeared posthumously.[23]
Hofmann was born in Prague and received a degree in medicine from
the University of Prague. He lived and taught in Innsbruck, Austria,
from 1869 to 1875 at which time he became a professor in Vienna.
His textbook referred to German and Austrian laws. The publication

---

[19] Quoted in Erwin H. Ackerknecht, "Legal Medicine Becomes a Modern Science
(19th Century)," *Ciba Symposia* 11 (1949-1951): 1304.

[20] Nemec, *Highlights in Medicolegal Relations*, 73.

[21] Johann Ludwig Casper, *A Handbook of the Practice of Forensic Medicine,
Based upon Personal Experience*, transl. from the 3rd ed. of the original by Geo.
W. Balfour, 4 vols. (London: New Sydenham Society, 1861-1865).

[22] Ludwig Johann Casper, *Practisches Handbuch der Gerichtlichen Medizin*,
Zweiter Band (Biologischer Theil) (Berlin: August Hirschwald, 1858), 31. Editions:
1: 1857-1858; 3: 1860; 5: 1871 (ed. by Liman); 6: 1876 (ed. by Liman); 8: 1889
(ed. by Liman); 9: 1905 (ed. by Schmidtmann).

[23] Eduard Ritter von Hofmann, *Lehrbuch der gerichtlichen Medicin: Mit
besonderer Berücksichtigung der österreichischen und deutschen Gesetzgebung*
(Vienna: Urban & Schwarzenberg, 1878). Editions: 1: 1878; 2: 1881; 3: 1883-
1884; 4: 1887; 5: 1891; 6: 1893; 7: 1895; 8: 1898; 9: 1909 (ed. by Kolisko); 10:
1919-1923 (ed. by Haberda); 11: 1927 (ed. by Haberda).

of the eighth edition in 1898 coincided with his death,[24] just before the German legislation mandated changes in the practice of forensic medicine. On September 16, 1899, Prussian laws for district medical officers changed; on January 1, 1900, a new German civil code was enacted; and new examination regulations were required for physicians at German universities after May 18, 1901. In decisive ways, then, the eighth edition marked the end of German forensic medicine in the nineteenth century. The death of Hofmann, the legal changes, and the eighth edition of Hofmann's textbook delineate the terminal point of this study.[25]

Although these textbooks by Henke, Caspar, and Hofmann are major sources, numerous other books enrich the analysis. Based on the insight of Crawford that "the history of forensic medicine is a story of medicalization,"[26] the following section examines a wide variety of textbooks to describe their ideas about rape as a medical phenomenon.

Ideas about Rape

"Men have become more moral and women perhaps more yielding, which is why in our time examples of rape are so rare, after having caused forensic doctors so much trouble," the forensic scientist Wolfgang F. W. Klose wrote in 1814.[27] However, in 1861, subsuming rape under the general category of "crimes against morality," another

---

[24] For further information see B. Davis, "A History of Forensic Medicine," *Medicolegal Journal* 53 (1985): 9-23; Richard O. Myers, "Famous Forensic Scientists: 7—Eduard Ritter von Hofmann (1837-1897)," *Medicine, Science and the Law* 3, no. 1 (October 1962): 18-24; Fritz Reuter, *Geschichte der Wiener Lehrkanzel für gerichtliche Medizin von 1804-1954*, Beiträge zur Gerichtlichen Medizin, XIX-Supplement (Vienna: Franz Deuticke, 1954); Leopold Schönbauer, *Das Medizinische Wien: Geschichte, Werden, Würdigung*, 2. umgearbeitete und erweiterte Auflage (Vienna: Urban & Schwarzenberg, 1947).

[25] A. Schmidtmann, ed., *Handbuch der Gerichtlichen Medizin*, 9. Auflage des Casper-Limanschen Handbuches, vol. 1 (Berlin: August Hirschwald, 1905), iii.

[26] Crawford, "Medicine and the Law," 1620. See also Meyer-Knees, *Verführung*, 124-28.

[27] Klose, *System*, 269: "Die Männer sind gesitteter und die Weiber vielleicht nachgiebiger geworden, daher in unsern Tagen die Seltenheit der Beispiele von Nothzucht, die ehemals den gerichtlichen Physikern so viel zu schaffen machte." See also Albert Meckel, *Lehrbuch der gerichtlichen Medicin* (Halle: C. F. Schimmelpfennig, 1821), 451: "Die Klagen der Nothzucht waren ehemals weit häufiger als jetzt."

forensic scholar, I. H. Schürmayer, observed: "Offences against morality have significantly increased in recent times. . . ."[28] Twenty years later, the forensic scholar Carl Liman exclaimed: "Everywhere crimes against morality are increasing shockingly."[29]

These quotations demonstrate that the perception of rape underwent an enormous change during the nineteenth century. While forensic scholars initially considered rape a problem of the past, they later acknowledged the growing incidence of rape in German society. Explanations are more extensive during the second half of the century than they were in the first. However, basic ideas about rape remained remarkably stable and permanent, as the ensuing discussions demonstrate. They identify five ways in which forensic scholars conceptualized the issue.

Rape as Illegal Intercourse

Many textbooks discussed rape in chapters alongside other sexual matters. Instead of being treated as a separate issue, rape was juxtaposed to "pederasty,"[30] lesbianism, sodomy, bestiality, and necrophilia.[31] All these issues were classified under the rubric "illegal intercourse." Even in textbooks that attempted to separate rape from other sexual issues,[32] chapter headings classified it as one among other

---

[28] Ignaz Heinrich Schürmayer, *Lehrbuch der Gerichtlichen Medicin*, 3. gänzlich umgearbeitete und verbesserte Auflage (Erlangen: Ferdinand Enke, 1861), 356: "Die Vergehen gegen die Sittlichkeit haben sich in neuerer Zeit bedeutend vermehrt . . . ."

[29] Johann Ludwig Casper, *Practisches Handbuch der Gerichtlichen Medicin*, neu bearbeitet und vermehrt von Carl Liman, Erster Band (Biologischer Theil), 5. Auflage (Berlin: August Hirschwald, 1871), 115: "Überall machen sich die Verbrechen gegen die Sittlichkeit in erschreckender Progression geltend."

[30] Quotation marks are used with the term "pederasty" because at that time it covered what the term "homosexuality" describes today. For a history of the terminology see Jonathan Katz, *The Invention of Heterosexuality* (New York: Dutton, 1995).

[31] For a similar observation on this point from a historical-legal perspective see Eveline Teufert, *Notzucht und sexuelle Nötigung: Ein Beitrag zur Kriminologie und Kriminalistik der Sexualfreiheitsdelikte unter Berücksichtigung der Geschichte und der geltenden strafrechtlichen Regelung*, Kriminalwissenschaftliche Abhandlung, vol. 14 (Lübeck: Max Schmidt-Römhild, 1980), 33f.

[32] See Müller, *Entwurf*; Theodor G. A. Roose, *Grundriss medizinisch-gerichtlicher Vorlesungen* (Frankfurt/Main: Wilmans, 1802); Johann A. H. Nicolai, *Handbuch der gerichtlichen Medicin nach dem gegenwärtigen Standpunkt dieser Wissenschaft für Aerzte und Criminalisten* (Berlin: August Hirschwald, 1841); Johannes B. Friedrich, *Handbuch der Gerichtsaerztlichen Praxis, mit Einschluss der gerichtlichen Veterinärkunde*, 2 vols. (Regensburg: G. J. Munz, 1843-1844).

"devious" forms of intercourse. Henke's textbook presented a discussion on rape in the chapter entitled "Examinations about Unclear Sexual Conditions."[33] Christian F. L. Wildberg's textbook used the title "Examinations with Regard to Intercourse."[34] Johann D. Metzger proposed "Illegal Intercourse."[35] Franz von Ney wrote "On Rape and Other Cases of Vice."[36] Ferdinand Hauska's textbook employed the chapter title "Prohibited Ways to Satisfy the Sexual Urge."[37] J. Maschka treated rape in the chapter "Signs of Virginity and Illegal Satisfaction of the Sexual Urge."[38]

A close analysis of several forensic textbooks uncovers the continuous process in which rape was merged with other forms of "illegal intercourse." The first edition of Henke's work is a good example.[39] A chapter entitled "Examinations Concerning Unclear Sexual Conditions" contained a section "About Illegal and Unnatural Intercourse §174-182." The section discusses rape along with "pederasty," sodomy, lesbianism, and bestiality. For Henke rape was not an issue unto itself; it belonged with "unnatural intercourses." The last edition of his work seemed to treat rape as a single issue in a section entitled "About

---

[33] Henke, *Lehrbuch*, 1859, 133: "Untersuchungen über zweifelhafte Geschlechtsverhältnisse."

[34] Christian F. L. Wildberg, *Handbuch der gerichtlichen Arzneywissenschaft zur Grundlage bey akademischen Vorlesungen und zum Gebrauche für ausübende gerichtliche Aerzte* (Berlin: W. Dieterici, 1812), 102: "Von den Untersuchungen in Hinsicht des Beyschlafes."

[35] Johann D. Metzger, *Kurzgefasstes System der gerichtlichen Arzneywissenschaft*, nach dem Todte des Verfassers revidirt, verbessert, mit den nöthigen Zusätzen und einem Register versehen von Dr. Christian Gottfried Gruner, 4. verbesserte und vermehrte Ausgabe (Königsberg/Leipzig: August Wilhelm Unzer, 1814), 457: "Gesetzwidriger Beyschlaf." Editions: 1: 1793; 2: 1798; 3: 1805.

[36] Franz von Ney, *Systematisches Handbuch der gerichtsarzneilichen Wissenschaft mit besonderer Berücksichtigung der Erhebung des Thatbestandes im Straf- und Civilverfahren für Aerzte, Wundärzte, dann Justiz- und politische Beamte und Advokaten in den k.k. Staaten, nebst einem Anhange über den Geschäftsstyl* (Vienna: Mörschner's Witwe & W. Bianchi, 1845), 77: "Von der Nothzucht und anderen Unzuchtsfällen."

[37] Ferdinand Hauska, *Compendium der gerichtlichen Arzneikunde*, 2. umgearbeitete Auflage (Wien: Braumüller, 1869), 11: "Verbotene Arten der Befriedigung des Geschlechtstriebes."

[38] J. Maschka, *Handbuch der Gerichtlichen Medicin*, vol. 3 (Tübingen: H. Laupp, 1882), 88: "Zeichen der Jungfrauschaft und gesetzwidrige Befriedigung des Geschlechtstriebes."

[39] Henke, *Lehrbuch*, 1812.

Rape §181-185,"[40] which was distinct from the section entitled "Unnatural Intercourse §186-188." Both sections remained, however, in the chapter entitled "About Illegal and Unnatural Intercourse." Thus rape continued to appear with these other issues. A textbook by G. H. Masius manifested the same design.[41] In a chapter entitled "About Illegal Intercourse," the discussion of rape follows one about virginity and precedes another about sodomy. Like Henke, Masius did not treat rape as an issue unto itself, but rather as one form of illegal intercourse.

Casper displayed an intriguing change on this classification.[42] In a section entitled "Contested Sexual Conditions," he treated three issues: "Contested Capability of Reproduction," "Contested Loss of Virginity," and "Contested Perverse Vice." At first glance, rape appears to be missing because it is not explicitly mentioned. A closer look, however, shows that Casper discussed rape in the section about virginity. In addition, he placed a reference about rape within a discussion of homosexuality entitled "Comparison of Pederasty to Rape." Thus he linked rape with virginity and "pederasty," although this connection does not appear in the titles of the chapters. All nineteenth-century editions of his textbook reflect this pattern. As in Henke and Masius, Casper characterized rape as "illegal and unnatural intercourse."

Hofmann's famous textbook continued this trend. He too considered rape as one form of "illegal and unnatural intercourse."[43] The chapter entitled "The Illegal Satisfaction of the Sexual Urge" included a section on "perverse vice," and linked rape to all the other forms of illegal intercourse. Hermann Kornfeld took an even more extreme position.[44] In his textbook no subdivisions are included in the chapter entitled "Examinations after Attacks against Morality." It interweaves comments about rape and "pederasty" as indecent practices and evaluations of homosexual intercourse with descriptions of forced hetero-

---

[40] Ibid, 1859.

[41] G. H. Masius, *Lehrbuch der gerichtlichen Arzneikunde für Rechtsgelehrte*, Ersther Theil: *Propädeutik zur gerichtlichen Arzneikunde*, zweite, sehr vermehrte und verbesserte Ausgabe (Altonau: Johann Friedrich Hammerich, 1812).

[42] Casper, *Practisches Handbuch*, 1858.

[43] Hofmann, *Lehrbuch der gerichtlichen Medicin*, 1878.

[44] Hermann Kornfeld, *Handbuch der gerichtlichen Medicin in Beziehung zu der Gesetzgebung Deutschlands und des Auslandes, nebst einem Anhange enthaltend die einschlägigen Gesetze und Verordnungen Deutschlands, Oesterreichs und Frankreichs* (Stuttgart: Ferdinand Enke, 1884).

sexual intercourse. Not differentiating between rape and "pederasty," Kornfeld viewed them as aspects of a single issue, namely attacks against morality. His view is but another example of the overall stance of nineteenth-century forensic scholars. Like biblical commentaries, forensic textbooks subsumed rape within a broader category.

Rape and Distrust

Another way scholarly and professional writers handled the issue of rape was to distrust a woman's testimony. Henke wrote:

> Wegen der sehr häufig falschen Anklagen über Nothzucht hat man zuvörderst die Frage aufgeworfen: Ob die Nothzucht überall möglich sei?[45]

> Because of frequently false accusations of rape, one asks above all: Is rape possible everywhere?

This statement of profound distrust followed a discussion about the possibility of rape between a strong man and an equally strong and healthy woman. Henke stated that such a woman could not be raped.[46] Similarly, Christian F. L. Wildberg argued:

> Ein Stuprum violentum consummatum einer erwachsenen, gesunden, gleich starken, sich ganz bewussten, und zumal im jungfräulichen Zustande sich befindenden Person, von einem einzelnen Manne durch blosse Körperkraft, ist mit fast allen Lehrern der gerichtlichen Arzeneywissenschaft wohl allerdings für unmöglich zu halten.[47]

---

[45] Henke, *Lehrbuch*, 1859, 128.

[46] Ibid., 128.

[47] Wildberg, *Handbuch*, 115. See also Ernst Buchner, *Lehrbuch der Gerichtlichen Medicin für Aerzte und Juristen* (Munich: J. A. Finsterlin, 1867), 194; Friedreich, *Handbuch*, II, 1843, 283f; Klose, *System*, 270; Adolph Lion, *Taschenbuch der gerichtlichen Medicin nach dem neuesten Standpunkt der Wissenschaft und der Gesetzgebungen Deutschlands zum Gebrauche für Aerzte und Juristen* (Erlangen: Ferdinand Enke, 1861), 130; G. H. Masius, *Handbuch der gerichtlichen Arzneiwissenschaft: Zum Gebrauche für gerichtliche Ärzte und Rechtsgelehrte*, Erster Band, Erste Abtheilung, 3d ed. (Stendahl: Franzen & Grosse, 1821), 246; Meckel, *Lehrbuch*, 469; J. D. Metzger, *System der gerichtlichen Arzneywissenschaft*, nach dem Tode des Verfassers verbessert und mit Zusätzen versehen von Dr. Christian Gottfried Gruner, erweitert und berichtigt von Wilhelm Hermann Georg Remer, 5th ed. (Königsberg/ Leipzig:A. W. Unzer, 1820), 469; Johann F. Niemann, *Handbuch der Staats-Arzneywissenschaft und staatsärztlichen Veterinärkunde nach alphabetischer Ordnung für Aerzte, Medicinalpolizei-Beamte und Richter,*

A rape of a grown-up, equally strong, completely conscious, and especially virginal person done by a single man only through physical strength is indeed to be considered as impossible according to almost all teachers of forensic medicine.

Forensic investigators dismissed a rape accusation if in their judgment the woman was able to fight off her attacker. The perception of the expert was valued above the testimony of the raped woman. Forensic scientists provided detailed instructions on a woman's method for resisting: with equal physical strength as well as with her "natural" weapons—her hands and especially her nails. Thus Johannes B. Friedreich proposed:

Wenn demnach ein erwachsenes, gesundes und mässig starkes Frauenzimmer behauptet, durch körperliche Gewalt von einem einzelnen Manne genothzüchtigt zu seyn, so verdient es keinen Glauben.[48]

If, therefore, a grown-up, healthy, and moderately strong woman claims to have been raped by a single man because of his physical strength, this statement does not deserve credence.

The forensic world profoundly distrusted women who claimed that they had been raped. The assumption that "for every ten accusations of rape nine might easily be wrong"[49] fueled suspicion against raped women and supported rapists.

Throughout the first half of that century forensic doctors contested the rape charges of women. Dismissing them as profit-seeking strategies or ungrounded accusations,[50] scholar after scholar concluded that,

---

2 vols. (Leipzig: J. Ambrosius Barth, 1813), 109f; Roose, *Grundriss*, 67; Johann A. Schmidtmüller, *Handbuch der Staatsarzneykunde zu Vorlesungen und zum Gebrauche für Bezirksärzte, Polizei-und Justizbeamte* (Landshut: Krüll, 1804), 207; Friedrich J. Siebenhaar, *Enzyklopädisches Handbuch der gerichtlichen Arzneikunde für Aerzte und Rechtsgelehrte*, in Verbindung mit Friedr. Erdm. Flachs et al., 2. Band (Leipzig: Engelmann, 1840), 306; Casper Jacob E. von Siebold, *Lehrbuch der gerichtlichen Medicin: Zur Grundlage bei academischen Vorlesungen und zum Gebrauch für gerichtliche Aerzte und Rechtsgelehrte* (Berlin: T. Chr. F. Enslin, 1847), 108. For a different view see Ludwig J. K. Mende, *Ausführliches Handbuch der gerichtlichen Medizin für Gesetzgeber, Rechtsgelehrte, Aerzte und Wundärzte*, vol. 4 (Leipzig: Dyk, 1826), 480f.

[48] Friedreich, *Handbuch*, II, 1843, 285; see also Masius, *Handbuch*, 246.

[49] Henke, *Lehrbuch*, 1859, 129.

[50] Metzger, *System*, 466.

according to his observations, a woman equal in strength to a man could not be raped by him.[51] Read in this context, the suggestion of Carl G. L. Bergmann was not surprising:

> Die Klagen über dergleichen Verbrechen sind so häufig unbegründet, daß es nicht ohne Interesse sein würde, durch statistische Bearbeitung den Grad von Zweifel zu bestimmen, mit welchem im Allgemeinen eine solche Klage angenommen werden müßte.[52]

> Complaints about such crimes are so often unfounded that it would be interesting to determine statistically the degree of doubt with which such a complaint should generally be evaluated.

Bergmann proposed to introduce mathematical tools for evaluating a woman's complaint so that forensic scholars would not have to rely on her word.

Lacking such measurements, some scholars offered alternatives to establish the truth of the accusation. The forensic doctor Adolph Lion recommended the following procedure:

> Sehr wesentlich, wie bei allen geschlechtlichen Untersuchungen ist hier die Art und Weise, wie der Gerichtsarzt physiologisch seine Untersuchung anstellt. Er lasse sich den Vorgang genau erzählen, achte auf Ausdrücke, Moralität und Benehmen, sowohl des Kindes als der Angehörigen und derer, die sonst ein Interesse zu haben vermeinen, suche besonders Widersprüche und unwahrscheinliche Angaben zu ermitteln, und er wird im Zusammenhang mit dem physischen Befunde in der Regel die Wahrheit ermitteln. Wenn Lehrer, Vorsteher von Anstalten, Aerzte, Beamte überhaupt beschuldigt werden, sei man besonders auf seiner Hut.[53]

> As with all sexual examinations, what is essential here is the way in which the forensic physician carries out his examination. He should be told the exact events of the rape. He should pay attention to the expressions, morality, and behavior both of the child and the relatives and of those who are believed to have an interest. He should especially search for contradictions and improbable descriptions. Together with the physical finding, he will usually detect the truth. If teachers, directors of institutions, physicians, or officials are accused, a doctor should be particularly on his guard.

---

[51] Cf. Siebold, *Lehrbuch*, 1-3; Metzger, *System*, 27.

[52] Carl G. L. Ch. Bergmann, *Lehrbuch der Medicina forensis für Juristen* (Braunschweig: Vieweg, 1846), 370.

[53] Lion, *Taschenbuch*, 132.

Concomitant with these measures, Masius also proposed to look at the woman's personality, her way of life, and educational background:

> In vorkommenden Fällen muss dabey vorzüglich auf das weibliche Individuum gesehen, und das Temperament, die Erziehung, und Lebensart desselben wohl erwogen werden. Das Temperament des sonst nicht berüchtigten Frauenzimmers sollte überhaupt bey Beurtheilung eines Stupri consummati stets berücksichtigt werden.[54]

> In occuring cases one must focus primarily on the female individual and consider the temperament, education, and way of life. The temperament of a woman not known to be notorious should indeed always be considered when one evaluates a stupri consummati.

Forensic scholars scrutinized the behavior of a woman who filed a rape charge. Describing the task of the physician, J. Maschka illuminated further her paradoxical situation:

> Das ganze Verhalten und Benehmen der Person, die Art und Weise wie sie den Hergang erzählt und sich hierbei ausdrückt, geben, wenn man nur einige Erfahrung und Uebung hat, oft unwillkürlich, ich möchte fast sagen, fast instinktmässig, einen ziemlich sicheren Anhaltspunkt zur Bestimmung, ob Wahrheit gesprochen oder falsche Angaben gemacht werden. Nur muß man sich hüten, allzugrosse Prüderie und Verschämtheit stets für die Wahrheit zu halten, indem gerade die Erfahrung lehrt, dass unschuldige Frauenspersonen sich sehr bescheiden benehmen und sich leicht in die vorzunehmende Untersuchung fügen, während unzüchtige und dem Dienste der Venus ergebene Personen bei solchen Gelegenheiten sich scheinbar sträuben und Hindernisse darbieten . . . . Das oft mit empörender Frechheit verbundene oder wie eine eingelernte Aufgabe erfolgende Herrecitieren des angeblichen Sachverhaltes lässt häufig auf hochgradige moralische Verkommenheit oder auf ein Eingelerntsein der angegebenen Daten schliessen.[55]

> The entire behavior and conduct of a person, the way in which she describes the event and how she expresses it, give, if one has some experience and practice, almost instinctively a relatively certain indication to decide if truth has been spoken or false descriptions have been made. One has to be careful

---

[54] Masius, *Lehrbuch*, 1812, 248.

[55] Maschka, *Handbuch*, III, 132-33. See also Bergmann, *Lehrbuch*, 370. 374; Buchner, *Lehrbuch*, 196; Henke, *Lehrbuch*, 1812, 101; Hofmann, *Lehrbuch*, 1878, 147; Lion, *Taschenbuch*, 132; Müller, *Entwurf*, 121; Wilhelm Pichler, *Die gerichtliche Medizin, nach dem heutigen Standpunkte der Medizin und der Gesetzgebung in ihren Umrissen dargestellt* (Vienna: Wallishausser, 1861), 25; Siebenhaar, *Enzyklopädisches Handbuch*, II, 1844, 308ff.

not to consider too much prudery and bashfulness for the truth because experience teaches that innocent women behave very modestly and comply easily
with the examination that will be performed. However, obscene persons and
those who have submitted to serve Venus apparently resist and invent ob-
stacles . . . . Often combined with outrageous freshness and like a learned
assignment, the recitation of the alleged facts frequently suggests extreme
immorality or the memorization of the alleged data.

In this point of view, no matter what a raped woman told the physician, her credibility was at risk. If she behaved modestly and prudishly,
the physician concluded that she had lied. If she objected to the gyne-
cological examination, the physician concluded that she was trying to
hide her immoral habits. The doctor's power allowed him to reject her
claim on the basis of his own "instinct," a truly vague standard. Repeatedly, forensic physicians were encouraged to be suspicious about
women's complaints about rape. Openly distrustful, they scrutinized
not only the woman's body but also her whole personality and background. A raped woman thus could not project a trustworthy image
during the examination. In the context of assumed scientific objectivity, the medical world encouraged distrust of rape claims. This stance
echoes positions adopted by biblical critics who dismissed the brothers of the raped woman and tended to protect the rapist.

Rape as Libido
Although most forensic scholars concluded that a strong man could
not rape an equally strong woman, others rejected that view. Nicolai[56]
and Schürmeyer[57] claimed that a strong man could rape an equally
strong and healthy woman. Even Wildberg, who in 1812 defended the
impossibility of a rape involving equally strong participants, later admitted its possibility:

> Dass eine gewaltsame oder betrügliche Nothzucht einer erwachsenen gesunden
> sich bewussten Person durch *einen* Mann allein vollkommen vollbracht sein
> kann, und dass bei derselben Empfängnis und Schwängerung möglich ist,
> darf er nicht allemal geradezu läugnen. Denn es kann, wenn die männliche
> Ruthe alles weiblichen Widerstrebens ungeachtet bis an oder in die Scheide
> gelangt, gerade zur Zeit der gänzlichen Erschöpfung der Kräfte des Weibes
> die wider Willen der Person dennoch geschehene örtliche wollüstige Reizung

---

[56] Nicolai, *Handbuch,* 162. On the issue of libido in forensic medicine see also
Meyer-Knees, *Verführung,* 160.
[57] Schürmayer, *Lehrbuch,* II, 1854, 332.

der Geschlechtstheile den höchsten, alle Widerstandsfähigkeit völlig lähmenden Grad erreicht haben, und dann gar wohl eine Schwängerung möglich werden.[58]

That a violent or fraudulent rape of a grown-up, healthy, conscious person can be completed by *one* man alone and that this makes possible conception and impregnation should not always be denied. Because it may be, when the male penis reaches the vagina despite all female resistance exactly at the time of the complete exhaustion of the woman's strength, that the lewd stimulation of the genitals done against the will of the person achieves its highest degree, paralyzing all her power of resistance and then making an impregnation possible.

The question was whether the physical stimulation of a woman forced her psychologically to give in and consent to the forced sexual intercourse. Forensic scholars imagined that her libido took over so extensively that the woman was not raped physically. Her body supposedly enjoyed the physical manipulations so that her willpower collapsed. She was raped psychologically though not physically because her body enjoyed the activity. Even Friedreich, for whom rape between equally strong participants remained impossible, stressed the force of the libido in overpowering the will of a woman. In his textbook he wrote:

Es ist möglich, dass bei einem Frauenzimmer, welches anfangs durchaus nicht in den Beischlaf gewilligt und sich jedem Versuche dazu ernstlich widersetzt hat, dennoch zuletzt durch die Verführungsmanipulationen und Liebkosungen des Mannes die Sinnlichkeit und der Geschlechtstrieb so erregt wird, dass es sich dann ohne ferneren Widerstand der Umarmung des Mannes vollständig hingiebt. Vom physischen Gesichtspunkte ausgegangen, scheint zwar hier zuletzt keine Nothzucht begangen worden zu seyn: allein es ist hier an die Stelle des körperlichen Zwanges der psychische getreten und es ist hier das weibliche Individuum durch Erregung eines hohen Grades seines Geschlechtstriebes in einen passiven und somit auch gewissermassen willenslosen Zustand versetzt, und demnach doch genothzüchtigt worden.[59]

It is possible that seduction and fondling arouse a woman's eroticism and libido, so that she will surrender to the man's embrace without further resistance although at first she really did not agree to the intercourse and seriously resisted any attempt. From a physical point of view no rape seems to have been committed. However, physical coercion is replaced by psychological

---

[58] Christian F. L. Wildberg, *Codex medico-forensis oder Inbegriff aller in gerichtlichen Fällen von den Gerichts-Aerzten zu beobachtenden Vorschriften*, neu bearbeitet (Leipzig: F. A. Brockhaus, 1849), 41f.

[59] Friedreich, *Handbuch*, II, 1844, 287.

coercion, and the female individual is put into a passive and almost will-less condition because of strong arousal, and thus she has been raped indeed.

Many scientists imagined that the movement of the penis sexually stimulated a woman despite her initial or continuous resistance. The forensic writer Johann A. Schmidtmüller thought that the libido of a woman was aroused despite her resistance, if the "fiery lover" immediately raped her a second time.[60] Masius stated that a rapist would take advantage when the libido overwhelmed the woman, a situation thus complicating the medical decision as to whether the intercourse was voluntary.[61] Klose imagined that even a "fiery girl who is unexperienced in physical love will easily . . . be enraptured by a certain degree of libido . . . especially if the sight of the rapist is concealed in the darkness of the night."[62]

The idea of the libido overwhelming a woman during a rape shows that these scholars viewed rape not as an attack on a woman's entire being but as a physically satisfying encounter between a man and a woman. Although forensic scholars considered the possibility of "psychological" rape, their case studies do not indicate that judicial decisions were based on that concept.[63]

This understanding of rape as libido derived from a particular view of nature. Friedreich exemplified the connection when he exclaimed:

> Die Natur hat den höchsten sinnlichen Reiz in das Zeugungsgeschäft gelegt und dem Zeugungstriebe eine grosse Kraft ertheilt. Die aufgeregte Geschlechtslust bemeistert sich des ganzen Individuums und in je höherem Grade dieses der Fall ist, desto eher durchbricht sie die Schranken, die ihr Zweck, die Erhaltung des Ganzen, vorgezeichnet hat.[64]

> Nature has put the highest sensual attraction into the procreative act and given great power to the procreative instinct. Aroused libido dominates the whole individual, and the more that happens, the more it breaks those boundaries which its purpose, the maintenance of the whole, has prescribed.

By regarding procreation and libido as unescapable facts of nature, Friedreich introduced the possibility of doubting that rape was a seri-

---

[60] Schmidtmüller, *Handbuch*, 209. See also Mende, *Ausführliches Handbuch*, IV, 479; Müller, *Entwurf*, 129f; Siebenhaar, *Enzyklopädisches Handbuch*, II, 1844, 307.

[61] Masius, *Handbuch*, I, 1821, 247f.

[62] Klose, *System*, 272-73.

[63] For a selection of case studies see Casper, *Practisches Handbuch*, II, 1858.

[64] Friedreich, *Handbuch*, II, 1844, 269.

ous transgression. He held that if men kept their libido within marriage, quarrels about seduction might occur, but rape could not. It occurred only when men failed to satisfy the libido within married life. In short, rape was part of the continuum of the libido. This view resonates with commentators who emphasize the love of Shechem. Much as love could overcome the rape in Genesis 34, so here the libido makes rape a pleasant experience for the woman.

Rape and Physical Maturity

When forensic scholars discussed the issue of rape, they usually referred to girls under the age of fourteen years.[65] Nineteenth-century German law codes were one reason for this restrictive understanding. Those codes judged any adult male sexual act with girls under the age of fourteen years as rape, with or without the consent of the girl.[66] Forensic scholars were, of course, aware of this fact but recognized that an alleged rapist might not know the age of the young woman. So in giving evidence to the court, they had to decide whether the girl seemed older than fourteen years. The skill to make such a judgment was assumed to be easy. Indeed, Paul Dittrich argued, "In many such cases it would also be easy for the layperson to judge the age of a girl."[67] If the accused claimed to have believed that the girl was older, forensic scientists freed him of the charge. Rape was punishable only

---

[65] See, for example, Joseph Bernt, *Beyträge zur gerichtlichen Arzneykunde für Ärzte, Wundärzte und Rechtsgelehrte*, vol. 1 (Vienna: C. Gerold, 1818), 71; Casper, *Practisches Handbuch*, I, 1871, 114; Henke, *Lehrbuch*, 1859, 129; Hauska, *Compendium*, 11; Klose, *System*, 271; Lion, *Taschenbuch*, 130; Maschka, *Handbuch*, 101. 102; Masius, *Lehrbuch*, 1812, 249, 250f; Meckel, *Lehrbuch*, 469; Mende, *Handbuch*, IV, 477f; Metzger, *System*, 470; Ney, *Handbuch*, 78, 84; Nicolai, *Handbuch*, 161. 166; Pichler, *Die gerichtliche Medizin*, 26. 28; Roose, *Grundriss*, 68; Schmidtmüller, *Handbuch*, 207, 208; Strassman, *Lehrbuch*, 151.

[66] For a quotation of the law codes see Friedrich Wilhelm Bocker, *Lehrbuch der gerichtlichen Medicin, mit Berücksichtigung der gesammten deutschen und rheinischen Gesetzgebung als Leitfaden zu seinen Vorlesungen und zum Gebrauche für Aerzte und Juristen*, 2. sehr vermehrte und verbessert Auflage (Iserlohn: Badeker, 1857), 263-68; Hofmann, *Lehrbuch*, 1903, 94-95. For references to nineteenth-century French, English, and American laws concerning rape see Kornfeld, *Handbuch*, 418-19.

[67] Paul Dittrich, *Lehrbuch der gerichtlichen Medizin, mit Berücksichtigung der deutschen, österreichischen und bernischen Gesetzgebungen* (Leipzig: Thieme, 1900), 216: "In vielen solchen Fällen wird es auch dem Laien leicht fallen, sich ein Urtheil über das Alter eines Mädchens zu bilden."

"if the perpetrator knew or could have assumed that the female individual had not yet reached this age."[68]

Hofmann explained why the German and the Austrian law codes chose the age of fourteen even though female maturity was sometimes reached after that age:

> Das 14. Jahr wurde als Grenze gesetzt mit Rücksicht auf die Erfahrung, dass in unserm Klima die Geschlechtsreife um diese Zeit sich einstellt.[69]

> The limit of fourteen years was chosen because in our climate sexual maturity is reached around this time.

Forensic scholars cited geographic location and climate to explain the legal boundary of fourteen years. They were aware that physical maturity was reached at different ages in different countries, "earlier in warmer climates where the burning skies favor every vegetation . . . later in northern climates because of an environment that is less favorable for the vegetation."[70] Schürmayer discussed differences in maturity even more precisely:

> So erscheint auf den Inseln des griechischen Archipelagus der Monatsfluss schon im zehnten Jahre, während er in Manchester im 15. und in Göttingen im 16. Jahr, im Durchschnitte, zu Stande kommt.[71]

> Accordingly, on the islands of the Greek archipelago menstruation starts on average at ten years, while it usually occurs in Manchester at the age of fifteen and in Göttingen at the age of sixteen years.

Referring to climate and geography, forensic scholars maintained that girls sometimes looked older than they really were. That argument enabled them to ignore the age boundaries set by the law codes and to allow rapists to avoid conviction. A woman's physical maturity could be used to excuse rape. The elaborate concern about Dinah's age resembles the forensic debate.

Lost Virginity as a Sign of Rape
Since observations of nature provided the principles of forensic medicine,[72] physical evidence was ultimately what decided the validity of a

---

[68] Ibid., 216: "Wenn der Thäter wusste oder annehmen konnte, dass die Frauensperson dieses Alter noch nicht erreicht hat."

[69] Hofmann, Lehrbuch, 1903, 150.

[70] Friedreich, Handbuch, II, 1844, 253f.

[71] Schürmayer, Lehrbuch, 109.

[72] See Klose, System, 27; Masius, Handbuch, X; Schmidtmüller, Handbuch, 1; Siebold, Lehrbuch, 1-2. On virginity see also Meyer-Knees, Verführung, 131-40.

rape charge. Many textbooks testified to the involved complications to find such physical evidence. In 1821, Masius acknowledged that physical examinations were invalid for adult women:

Zur Ausmittelung der Wahrheit des Vorgehens einer beschuldigten Nothzucht wird von dem Richter in der Regel die Besichtigung der Geschlechtstheile des angeblich geschändeten Frauenzimmers verfügt. Durch dieselbe kann der Beweis der That aber keineswegs in allen Fällen mit Gewissheit geführet werden, vielmehr ist durch die ärztliche Dazwischenkunft häufig gar keine Aufklärung zu erhalten.[73]

For the determination of the event's truth the judge usually requires that the genitals of the allegedly raped woman are examined. The examination will, however, not result in the certainty of proving the deed in all cases; rather, in many cases the medical interference will bring no clarification at all.

This scepticism regarding the benefit of physical examinations in cases of rape is part of a broader discussion. Doctors questioned the possibility to collect physical signs on the genitals of young men and women. After lengthy debates scholars concluded that physical signs on male genitals are too transient to be identifiable. In 1843, Friedrich stated in a section "On Male Virginity"[74] that the determination of male virginity is impossible. Likewise L. Krahmer stated:

Die Veränderungen, welche das Zustandekommen der gewöhnlichen Geschlechtsverrichtung oder die Ausübung des Beischlafs beim Manne hervorruft, sind so vergänglich, dass sie in den gerichtsärztlichen Compendien gar nicht erwähnt zu werden pflegen.[75]

The changes that are caused by the realization of the sexual act or the practice of intercourse in men are so transient that they are usually not even mentioned in forensic textbooks.

The search for physical signs on male genitals turned obsolete. In cases of rape, therefore, forensic doctors determined only the physical

---

[73] Masius, *Handbuch*, 1821, 250.

[74] Friedreich, *Handbuch*, II, 1844, 261.

[75] L. Krahmer, *Handbuch der Gerichtlichen Medzin für Aerzte und Juristen*, 2. umgearbeitete Auflage (Braunschweig: C. A. Schwetschke, 1857), 285. See also Bernhard Brach, *Lehrbuch der gerichtlichen Medicin* (Cologne: F. C. Eisen, 1846), 629: "Wenn schon die Untersuchung der Jungferschaft Schwierigkeiten hat und deren Ausmittelung öfters nicht mit Gewissheit zu bewerkstelligen ist, so steht es noch misslicher um die Junggesellschaft, indem die Veränderungen, die durch den ersten Beischlaf am Körper des Mannes bewirkt werden, zu unbedeutend und zu wenig characteristisch sind."

strength of the alleged rapist in comparison to the woman's. They looked for the size of his gentials in relation to hers and for general physical signs that would indicate resistance from the woman.[76]

Forensic scholars also searched for physical signs at female genitals. After extensive physical examinations of sexually experienced women, physicians concluded that female adult genitals did not provide sufficient evidence. Siebold stated:

> Die Nothzucht an erwachsenen Frauenzimmern, deren Geschlechtstheile vor der That nicht mehr im jungfräulichen Zustande waren, hinterlässt an diesen selbst freilich keine Spuren.[77]

> Of course, rape leaves no traces on adult women whose genitals were not virginal before the deed.

Some scholars stated that forensic medicine would never be able to prove that a rape happened. At best, general physical signs would give evidence of a rape. For instance, Schürmayer claimed:

> Die gerichtliche Medicin vermag daher über die Frage: ob der jungfräuliche Zustand noch in seiner Integrität bestehe, keinen befriedigenden Aufschluss zu geben. Nur wo noch andere Umstände als Indicien bestehen, wie z.B. bei Nothzucht, lässt sich der durch Coitus verletzte jungfräuliche Zustand mit grösserer oder geringerer Wahrscheinlichkeit darthun.[78]

> Forensic medicine is therefore unable to answer satisfactorily the question whether the virginal condition consists in its integrity. Only where other signs exist as evidence, as, for example, with rape, the virginal condition injured by intercourse will be substantiated with more or less probability.

Since adult women were no longer virginal, rape could not destroy the hymen, the one physical sign considered reliable. Some scholars, how-

---

[76] See Friedreich, *Handbuch*, II, 1844, 290; Franz X. Güntner, *Handbuch der gerichtlichen Medizin für Mediziner, Rechtsgelehrte und Gerichtsärzte, mit Rücksichtsnahme auf die Schwurgerichte* (Regensburg: Manz, 1851), 50; Masius, *Handbuch*, 252f; Ignaz H. Schürmayer, *Theoretisch-practisches Lehrbuch der Gerichtlichen Medicin: Mit Berücksichtigung der neueren Gesetzgebungen des In- und Auslandes und des Verfahrens bei Schwurgerichten, für Ärzte und Juristen: Mit einem Anhange, enthaltend eine kurzgefasste practische Anleitung zu gerichtlichen Leichenobductionen* (Erlangen: Ferdinand Enke, 1850), 349; Siebenhaar, *Encyklopädisches Handbuch*, II, 309; Wildberg, *Codex medico-forensis*, 41; Wildberg, *Handbuch*, 117.

[77] Siebold, *Lehrbuch*, 110.

[78] Schürmayer, *Theoretisch-practisches Lehrbuch*, 2. Auflage, 1854, 63.

ever, questioned its reliability. Güntner represented this cautionary approach about the hymen as a sign for female virginity:

> Da in den §§. 110. 111. 112. gezeigt wurde, daß keine der angeführten Erscheinungen an und für sich, sondern nur deren Zusammenhang die Diagnose der Jungfrauschaft sichert . . . so ist es klar, daß nur mit der größten Vorsicht ein Gutachten, das über die Ehre einer Frauensperson entscheidend ist, abgegeben werden könne.[79]

> Since the paragraphs §§. 110. 111. 112 demonstrated that none of the mentioned signs secures the diagnosis of virginity but only a combination of those signs . . . it is clear that an expert opinion that decides upon the reputation of a woman can be submitted only with utmost care.

Güntner argued that in addition to the hymen other physical signs were required to settle a rape charge. Yet the majority of scholars relied on the existence or recent injury of the hymen in cases of rape. They ignored the cautious statements and maintained that only the genitals of a girl provided the necessary physical evidence. For example, Brach claimed:

> Nur bei Kindern und noch nicht mannbaren, oder wenigstens im Zustande der Jungfernschaft noch befindlichen Mädchen kann man erwarten, physische Merkmale der geschehenen Nothzucht an den Geschlechtstheilen aufzufinden und dies auch nur dann, wenn die Untersuchung nicht zu lange nach vollzogenem Beischlaf vorgenommen wird.[80]

> Only with children or not yet nubile girls who are still virginal can one expect to find physical signs on the genitals of the occurred rape and even then only when the examination is undertaken not too long after the performed intercourse.

The search for physical evidence led scholars to find such evidence only in virginal young women because only "traces of recent defloration" proved the charge.[81] They believed that "virginal individuals" showed definite signs of defloration after a rape. Therefore, the presence as well as the clear absence of a hymen made a rape accusation

---

[79] Güntner, *Handbuch*, 47; see also Brach, *Lehrbuch*, 626f; Friedreich, *Handbuch*, II, 1844, 260; Klose, *System*, XXIII; Roose, *Grundriss*, 95; Schmidtmüller, *Handbuch*, 203.

[80] Brach, *Lehrbuch*, 630; see also Bocker, *Lehrbuch*, 270; Güntner, *Handbuch*, 50; Henke, *Lehrbuch*, 1859, 130; Schmidtmüller, *Handbuch*, 208;

[81] Bocker, *Lehrbuch*, 269.

invalid.[82] Since the 1850s textbooks included numerous drawings of the hymen as the "objective sign." The form and features of a hymen helped doctors to determine a woman's sexual history and the possible truth of the rape charge.[83] Illustrating the diversity of hymens, the drawings were supposed to prevent physicians from misinterpreting injured, destroyed, or lacking hymens.[84] Hence, doctors assumed that young women and girls could become rape victims.

Rape statistics identified girls as the primary target of rape. In fact, statistics included in the textbooks listed girls as the largest number of rape cases since the 1850s.[85] And so, in 1895, Fritz Strassmann claimed that "attacks against morality" occurred rarely with women but often with children:

> Ueberhaupt sind es überwiegend Kinder, welche diesen Attentaten ausgesetzt sind, während Nothzucht an Erwachsenen geradezu als ein seltenes Object gerichtsärztlicher Thätigkeit bezeichnet werden muss.[86]

> Actually, mainly children are exposed to these attacks while rapes with adults have to be regarded as a rare object in forensic practice.

Because forensic scholars looked for physical evidence and found it in female children, adult women and men did not provide sufficient evidence. Adult women disappeared as rape victims. The burden of proof lays with female children. Recently lost virginity became, therefore, a central sign of rape.

* * * * * * * * *

Forensic medical textbooks in nineteenth-century Germany contained five basic ideas about rape.

1) They categorized rape as one form of illegal intercourse.
2) They encouraged distrust of rape claims.
3) They characterized rape as the result of the libido.

---

[82] See, for example, Kornfeld, *Handbuch*, 420; Hofmann, *Lehrbuch*, 1891, 103.

[83] For example, Dittrich, *Lehrbuch*, 200.

[84] Fritz Strassman, *Lehrbuch der gerichtlichen Medicin*, mit 78 in den Text eingedruckten Abbildungen und einer Tafel in Farbendruck (Stuttgart: Ferdinand Enke, 1895), 86-102.

[85] Schmidtmann, *Handbuch*, 171f.

[86] Strassmann, *Lehrbuch*, 76.

4) They discussed the relationship between rape and physical maturity.
5) They regarded lost virginity as the sign of rape. In varying ways and degrees all five eradicated a rape accusation by a woman.

Moreover, all five considered the woman the main bearer of physical evidence and placed on her the presumed responsibility for the alleged rape. The textbooks encouraged physicians to distrust a woman's claim to have been raped. A specific procedure for examining a raped woman was invented to elicit the truth of a rape charge. In each area one detected links of various sorts between these ideas and ideas prevalent in the biblical commentaries of the same century.

Summary

Without acknowledging directly each other's discourse, biblical and forensic medicine scholars of the nineteenth century evinced comparable ideas on the topic of rape. The first idea maintained that rape is not a topic in its own right. Biblical commentaries omitted explicit discussions of the rape. Frequently, chapter headings do not refer to it and expositions do not consider it. Forensic textbooks considered rape a subcategory of illegal intercourse, which included homosexuality, bestiality, and necrophilia.

The second idea about rape showed the bias of scholarly authorities for the male perspective. Biblical commentaries condemned the brothers and sympathized with Shechem and Jacob. In both literatures rape became another opportunity for male bonding against the woman and those who sided with her. Forensic textbooks distrusted a raped woman, claiming she may have invented the rape and falsely accused the man. Physical examinations and evaluations of her speech, behavior, and background were all used against her.

The third idea considered rape an experience of love and libido on the part of the rapist and also the woman. Many biblical critics defined rape as love by taking refuge in textual ambiguity. Love tamed rape into a pleasurable experience, appropriately leading to marriage. For that reason, these scholars stressed the marriage proposal as the solution for the "hasty" behavior of Shechem. Forensic scholars, in effect, echoed this idea. Although they evaluated the sexual drive of the rapist as an understandable factor that needed some redirection, they allowed the libido of the woman to minimize the rape. To the detriment of the woman, rape emerged as part of the continuum of libido. In forensic medicine rape resulted from libido; in biblical commentaries love resulted from rape.

The fourth idea made rape dependent on the age of the woman. Both biblical commentaries and forensic medicine showed that the older the woman, the less credible she became in claiming to have been raped. Biblical commentators argued extensively about Dinah's age, although the biblical text never mentions her age. For many scholars, Dinah's alleged maturity relativized Shechem's rape. The debate about Dinah's age suggests the impact of cultural ideas upon biblical interpretations. Forensic texts explained this interest of biblical scholars to clarify the age of Dinah. Bound by German law codes, forensic writers established the age of fourteen as the age of maturity for a girl. If, however, a younger girl appeared to be fourteen years or older, the rape charge changed and the burden of proof disadvantaged the woman.

The fifth idea held that, by emphasizing other issues, biblical commentaries and forensic medicine diverted from the event of rape and its significance. Explanations of the story relied upon stereotypes to explain the rape as a regular custom of "Oriental despotism" and the fraternal response as alien to European morals but normal in Oriental society. Forensic textbooks took a different path of diversion. Since forensic scholars were primarily interested in deriving answers from observations of "nature," they focused their attention on the physical signs of virginity. Knowledge about physical changes in a woman's body after a rape became the basis for judging an accusation of rape. Description of these signs became increasingly detailed. Forensic medical textbooks included numerous drawings to clarify the physical characteristics of virginity, and rape became less and less the focus.

As evidenced in biblical commentaries and forensic textbooks, discourse on rape in nineteenth-century Germany did not develop from the perspective of the raped woman. At best, this discourse relied on "scientific" observation; at worst, it appropriated the perspective of the rapist. Although one might dismiss these ideas as the sad artifacts of history, the study of the contemporary period will challenge that viewpoint.

Chapter 5

Obfuscating Rape:
Interpretations from 1970 to 1997

Contemporary biblical scholars have employed various foci to interpret Genesis 34. With a few exceptions most of these interpretations have not emphasized the rape in the story, though they refer to it. The evaluation of those references shows the impact on what some feminists have called a Western "rape culture."

Unlike the analysis of nineteenth-century German commentaries, the study of contemporary interpretations cuts across boundaries of religion and nationality. And unlike the German nineteenth-century commentaries, contemporary scholarship appears in many different genres. Commentaries, monographs, journal articles, and essays address Genesis 34. Scholars from different religious backgrounds, mainly Protestant but also Catholic and Jewish, have diversified the debate. Scholars from Britain, France, Germany, Israel, and particularly the United States have contributed to the conversation. Consequently, a rich collection of interpretations has developed during the last three decades.

Ideas on Rape

Contemporary interpretations approach Genesis 34 from five directions, necessitating an examination with five parts. The first part, entitled "Focus on the Men," examines the emphasis on the male characters of the story. The second, "Source Criticism," analyzes ideas about rape found in interpretations that use this method. The third section, "Tribal History," studies interpretations that view the characters as personifications of tribes. The fourth, entitled "Xenophobia," deals with interpretations that debate the issue of integration and exclusion in ancient Israel. The fifth, entitled "Feminist Approaches," considers interpretations which claim that perspective. Analysis will show that all five of these categories marginalized the rape.

Focus on the Men

Several interpretations focus on the male characters: Jacob, or the brothers Simeon and Levi, or Shechem. Some readings present a combination of male characters as the main actors.

Jacob

One category of interpretation emphasizes Jacob. Entitled "Tragedy Comes to Jacob's Household," the exegesis of Gordon Talbot places Genesis 34 within the broader context of Jacob's return to Canaan.[1] Talbot evaluates the rape of Dinah as "one of the greatest heartbreaks of his [Jacob's] life."[2] He sympathizes with Jacob but blames Dinah for leaving the house and seeking companionship among the Canaanite women. Talbot writes, "One must ask why Dinah was seeking her circle of friends among the daughters of Shalem [sic]. Some level of compromise had taken over in the family of Jacob."[3] He accuses the brothers of forgetting "that vengeance is the Lord's."[4] Compassionately attending to Jacob's fears, Talbot rejects Jacob's children.

Gila Ramras-Rauch also emphasizes Jacob by reading Genesis 34 as a part of the Jacob cycle.[5] Though she asks whether the two acts of violence—the rape of Dinah and the revenge of the brothers—can be equated, nevertheless, she focuses on Jacob's reaction to the rape. "The main protagonist" is Jacob, and his silence represents "under-

---

[1] Gordon Talbot, *A Study of the Book of Genesis: An Introductory Commentary on All Fifty Chapters of Genesis* (Harrisburg, PA: Christian Publications, 1981). For a recent and short reference to Genesis 34 focused on Jacob see Karen Armstrong, *In the Beginning: A New Interpretation of Genesis* (New York: Knopf, 1996), 94-98.

[2] Talbot, *A Study of the Book of Genesis*, 206.

[3] Ibid., 207.

[4] Ibid., 208. Ronald S. Hendel focuses also on Jacob. Simultaneously he minimizes Genesis 34 as a small unit within "a series of loosely connected episodes" about Jacob's life, cf. *The Epic of the Patriarch: The Jacob Cycle and the Narrative Traditions of Canaan and Israel* (Atlanta: Scholars Press, 1987), 161.

[5] Gila Ramras-Rauch, "Fathers and Daughters: Two Biblical Narratives," in *Mappings of the Biblical Terrain: The Bible as Text*, ed. Vincent L. Tollers and John Maier (Cranbury, NJ: Associated University Presses, 1990), 158-69.

standable caution."[6] His motives are "vindicated." He is "cautious," but his sons are "unruly" and the Hivites are "deceitful."[7]

Similarly emphasizing the significance of Jacob, Naomi H. Rosenblatt and Joshua Horwitz read Genesis 34 as a story containing "a strong indictment of parents who forfeit their moral authority as family leaders."[8] Although these authors approach the book of Genesis psychologically, they do not treat the rape in chapter 34 as an issue worthy of psychological consideration. Interested in the role of parents in the lives of their children, Rosenblatt and Horwitz find contemporary parents and Jacob in a similar position: "Like many of us, Jacob displays more ambivalence than resolve about controlling his adult children's behavior." They speculate why Jacob acted passivlely and theorize "that both Jacob and his sons are acting partly in response to conflicts buried deep in their relationship."[9] "Jacob's anguish in fatherhood" contributes to a family conflict between father and sons in which the father fails.[10]

Another interpretation focuses on Jacob as one of "the descendants of Abraham." Devora Steinmetz proposes that Genesis 34 explains how Jacob's family becomes a nation. Despite his initial condemnation in chapter 34:30, Jacob later affirms the revenge of his sons (48:22). The change in his evaluation of the sons' revenge indicates to Steinmetz that Genesis 34 describes the beginning of the "acquisition of land, this time through conquest."[11] As the descendants of Abraham, Jacob and his family participate in the effort to return to the land. The rape of Dinah becomes a "necessary" ingredient in this effort to "complete" the sins of the Canaanites[12] so that the ancestor Jacob and his family continue "a destiny already in progress."[13]

---

[6] Ibid., 163f.

[7] Ibid., 164.

[8] Naomi H. Rosenblatt and Joshua Horwitz, "The Rape of Dinah: Humiliation and Retaliation," chap. in *Wrestling with Angels: What the First Family of Genesis Teaches Us about Our Spiritual Identity, Sexuality, and Personal Relationships* (New York: Delacorte, 1995), 310.

[9] Ibid., 311.

[10] Ibid., 312.

[11] Devora Steinmetz, *From Father to Son: Kinship, Conflict, Continuity in Genesis* (Louisville, KY: Westminster and Knox Press, 1991), 141.

[12] Ibid., 142.

[13] Ibid. For a different evaluation of Jacob's "life in Canaan" and cursing of his sons in Genesis 49:5-7 see John J. Davis, *Paradise to Prison: Studies in Genesis* (Grand Rapids, MI: Baker, 1975), 256-58.

Briefly discussing Genesis 34 in a study of the book of Numbers, Mary Douglas also focuses on Jacob.[14] Jacob's curse of Simeon and Levi in Genesis 49:5-7 serves to explain why Jacob "can never forgive their attack on Shechem" although Dinah's "harlotry could be forgiven."[15] Siding with Jacob against his sons, Douglas defends Shechem. The narrative demonstrates that "anyone who covenants to worship the God of Abraham, whether or not descended from Abraham, is not to be attacked as the men of Shechem, but treated as an honourable ally."[16] The brothers betrayed this rule which Jacob held dear even after the "seduction" of his daughter.[17] Douglas gives Jacob the authoritative voice; the rape becomes incidental.

Terence E. Fretheim regards the judgment made by Jacob as the key element in the narrative: "Perhaps most important, the sharp and unambiguous judgment (indeed, a curse!) by Jacob on the violence of Simeon and Levi must stand as the primary clue about how we should interpret this chapter (49:5-7)."[18] He claims that Jacob rejects the violence his sons inflicted on the "rapist and lover of Dinah" because they used "their sister's predicament as an excuse to perpetrate violence."[19] Their father, however, stressed "the effects of the violence for the larger issues of life and well-being for the *community*."[20]

This antipathy toward the brothers and the focus on Jacob originate from Fretheim's sympathy for Shechem. Fretheim declares that "Shechem proceeds to act in a way *atypical* of rapists: He clings to Dinah . . . loves her . . . and speaks to her heart. . . . The latter phrase *may* cause Dinah's positive response" [stress added].[21] "Many-faceted

---

[14] Mary Douglas, *In the Wilderness: The Doctrine of Defilement in the Book of Numbers* (Sheffield, UK: JSOT Press, 1993), 203-07.

[15] Ibid., 205.

[16] Ibid., 207.

[17] Douglas refers continuously to the seduction of Dinah without explaining the reasons for this terminological choice. For example, on p. 206 Douglas states that: "Dinah had been seduced." For an interpretation which ignores the rape and focuses on Jacob see Nehama Leibowitz, *Studies in Bereshit (Genesis) in the Context of Ancient and Modern Jewish Bible Commentary*, 2d rev. ed. (Jerusalem: Haomanim, 1974), 380-87.

[18] Terence E. Fretheim, "The Book of Genesis: Introduction, Commentary, and Reflections," in *The New Interpreter's Bible*, ed. Leander E. Keck, vol. 1 (Nashville: Abingdon Press, 1994), 577.

[19] Ibid., 578.

[20] Ibid., 581.

[21] Ibid., 577.

love" overrules rape,[22] so that "this turn of events shifts the reader's response to Shechem in more positive directions." "Love language" creates "sympathy for Shechem."[23] Furthermore, Shechem "seek(s) to make things right." He offers generously to marry Dinah although "such generosity was certainly not necessary." The marriage proposal suggests to Fretheim that "Shechem's offer was in Dinah's best interests" within the legal tradition of ancient Israel.

While Fretheim stresses Shechem's love and generosity, he describes Dinah's brothers as suspicious characters and finally unacceptable. "They use religion as a vehicle for their deception."[24] Fretheim sees Jacob struggling to overcome the threat of destruction brought by his sons. Thus, it is Jacob who "is in special need of divine protection."[25] Dinah and the rape recede in his discussion.

The Brothers Simeon and Levi

A second category of interpretation places the brothers in the leading role. Interpreting Genesis 34 in light of Bedouin law, Clinton Bailey considers the brothers to represent that law because "many aspects of biblical life . . . are similar to traditional Bedouin life as lived by most Bedouin . . . until the 1960s, and still lived there by some even now."[26] Bailey considers the "deceit and ruthlessness of Simeon and Levi's actions" as being reflected within "the logic of Bedouin ideas about law and justice."[27] Jacob, however, rejects his sons' "desert logic"[28] and curses them, so that Bailey "marvel[s] at the spiritual progress" of Jacob.[29]

Walter Russell Bowie also focuses on the brothers, claiming that Genesis 34 explains why their father cursed Simeon and Levi in Genesis 49:6-7. Although Bowie initially commends the brothers for their

---

[22] Ibid., 580.

[23] Ibid., 577.

[24] Ibid., 578.

[25] Ibid., 580.

[26] Clinton Bailey, "How Desert Culture Helps Us Understand the Bible," *Bible Review* (August 1991): 16. For a similar argument see Morris S. Seale, *The Desert Bible: Nomadic Tribal Culture and Old Testament Interpretation* (New York: St. Martin's, 1974), 130-31.

[27] Bailey, "How Desert Culture," 17.

[28] Ibid., 20.

[29] Ibid., 38.

"moral conscience,"[30] later he considers the revenge "worse than the original offense, more cruel, more hateful, and more ruinous."[31] The emphasis on the brothers illustrates their abominable character.

Bruce Vawter concentrates on the brothers; indeed, he strongly condemns them. In his view, Genesis 34 describes how the sons of Israel conquered the town of Shechem. Their action demonstrates their strong will, but "certainly nothing good could come from what his [Jacob's] sons have done."[32] Vawter censures the brothers only to dismiss them and their actions.

The commentator Clyde M. Woods regards the brothers as the main characters, thus entitling Genesis 34 "Jacob's Sons Avenge Dinah."[33] He regards the story as a "sordid chapter in the career of Jacob's family" in which the two sons "proudly defend their cruel savagery and remain impenitent." He is astonished that "scripture records the wrongs even of those in the covenant line."[34] Although the brothers "held to higher sexual ideals than the degenerate Canaanites,"[35] the focus on the brothers does not lead Woods to evaluate them sympathetically.

For those who might wonder about the story's purpose, Gordon J. Wenham explains that the rape of Dinah "only constitutes scene 1, which gives the background to the vengeance wrought by her brothers on her attacker."[36] Although "Shechem was quite wrong to rape her," this scholar holds that "Shechem was not your callous anonymous rapist, so dreaded in modern society, but an affectionate young man."[37]

---

[30] Walter Russell Bowie, "Genesis: Exposition," in *The Interpreter's Bible*, ed. George Buttrick, vol. 1 (Nashville: Abingdon Press, 1953, 26th printing 1980), 733. Although Bowie was a professor of homiletics rather than a biblical scholar, his exposition builds on the work of the biblical scholar Cuthbert A. Simpson, "Genesis," in *The Interpreter's Bible*, vol. 1, 723-38. Suggesting that "this [is a] story of how Simeon and Levi lost their rights" (p. 733), Simpson applies source criticism to interpret Genesis 34.

[31] Ibid., 736.

[32] Bruce Vawter, *On Genesis: A New Reading* (Garden City, NY: Doubleday, 1977), 360.

[33] Clyde M. Woods, *The Living Way Commentary on the Old Testament*, vol. 1: *Genesis-Exodus* (Shreveport: Lambert, 1972), 87.

[34] Ibid., 89.

[35] Ibid., 87.

[36] Gordon J. Wenham, *Word Biblical Commentary: Genesis 16-50*, vol. 2 (Dallas, TX: Word Books, 1994), 310.

[37] Ibid., 317.

In fact, "the Hivites appear to be very obliging, reasonable men."[38] But the sons are "undoubtedly the heroes of this story."[39] The events lead to the problematic relationship between the father and the sons, the "deepening of the rift between Jacob and his sons."[40] The ingredients in the conflict are "Dinah and the Hivites," the title of his interpretation despite the focus on the brothers.

Everett Fox considers "the vengefulness and brutality of Yaakov's sons" the prelude to the Joseph story. Genesis 34 presents "a somewhat ambiguous situation" because the "Canaanite sexual behavior is odious"[41] and "the putative heroes are not always heroic."[42] This interpretation highlights the brothers and their revenge; it says little about the rape itself.

Meir Sternberg also considers the brothers to be the leading characters. Unlike other interpreters, he esteems them highly. He maintains that the narrator "balances" the rape and the killing by providing a sympathetic description of the brothers. Although Sternberg makes peculiar claims, for example, that a rapist appears less "intense" if he rapes a woman after falling in love with her,[43] his sympathy for the brothers is rare among contemporary interpreters. The brothers receive positive attention as "victims"[44] "to elicit maximum sympathy" for them.[45]

---

[38] Ibid., 318.

[39] Ibid., 319. An essay on the development of the Levites focuses on the brothers, particularly on Levi, to argue for their importance. See Götz Schmitt, "Der Ursprung des Levitentums," *Zeitschrift für die alttestamentliche Wissenschaft* 94 (1982): 575-99.

[40] Wenham, *Word Biblical Commentary*, 318.

[41] Everett Fox, *In the Beginning: A New English Rendition of the Book of Genesis* (New York: Schocken, 1983), 137.

[42] Ibid., 139.

[43] Meir Sternberg, *The Poetics of Biblical Narrative: Ideological Literature and the Drama of Reading* (Bloomington: Indiana University Press, 1987), 447. For a popular collection of traditional Jewish views on Genesis 34 see Harvey J. Fields, *A Torah Commentary For Our Times*, vol. 1: *Genesis* (New York: UAHC Press, 1990), 80-90.

[44] Sternberg, *The Poetics of Biblical Narrative*, 446. Sternberg's sympathetic treatment of the brothers has been criticized by Amnon Shapira, "Be Silent: An Immoral Behavior?" *Beit Mikra* 39 (1994): 232-44. Shapira examines Genesis 34:5 to advocate a favorable evaluation of father Jacob in contrast to the brothers. For another criticism see the interpretation by Danna N. Fewell in the section below, entitled "Feminist Approaches."

[45] Sternberg, *The Poetics of Biblical Narrative*, 455.

Shechem

Several scholars concentrate on Shechem. Discussing marriage rituals
in the Bible, John H. Otwell observes that Shechem asks his father to
arrange the wedding against custom.[46] The fact that a rape preceded
the request for marriage does not prevent Otwell from viewing Shechem
as a legitimate bridegroom.

Calum M. Carmichael accents Shechem despite the initial claim
that Genesis 34 "is written up in such a way as to reveal a profound
tension of viewpoints between Jacob and his two sons."[47] Relating
Deuteronomic legislation (Deuteronomy 22:13-29) to narrative texts,[48]
Carmichael designates Genesis 34 as the "Shechem story." In it
Shechem gives "vent to his passion" and treats Dinah with "great
tenderness."[49] Dinah, writes Carmichael, must have given "some indication that she was willing." He explains that "she took it upon herself
to go out and visit the women of the area, and when Shechem encountered her, he, a prince, treated her with great tenderness." In
contrast to Dinah, the brothers disclose a "very high sexual standard,"[50]
which Deuteronomic law supports. Showing the brothers "high regard,"[51] the Deuteronomist concurs with them that Shechem treated
Dinah as a prostitute because he "enjoy[s] her without the formalities
of making arrangements with her father or guardian."[52] Premaritally
"seducing" Dinah,[53] Shechem gave the Deuteronomist reason to explore the consequences for such lacking restraint among Israelite men.[54]

Similarly, Stuart A. West, focuses on Shechem. Putting Genesis 34
within "the context of history," he claims that the story recalls the
"conquest of Shechem" as "a symbol for the future conquest of the

---

[46] John H. Otwell, *And Sarah Laughed: The Status of Woman in the Old
Testament* (Philadelphia: Westminster Press, 1977), 33, 37.

[47] Calum M. Carmichael, *Women, Law, and the Genesis Traditions* (Edinburgh:
Edinburgh University Press, 1979), 33.

[48] Ibid., 4. Carmichael maintains that the sources of the Deuteronomic legislation
did not arise from everyday life in ancient Israel but from the literary traditions. Thus
he examines the link between biblical law and literature.

[49] Ibid., 36, 45.

[50] Ibid., 42.

[51] Ibid., 48.

[52] Ibid., 38.

[53] Ibid.; see also pp. 41, 46.

[54] Ibid., 36.

land of Canaan."[55] Although West briefly mentions the other characters, only Shechem receives a full and positive evaluation. He "was
man enough to do the 'right' thing by offering to marry her,"[56] since
he was "both captivated by Dinah's beauty and troubled by his conscience,"[57] details that do not appear in the biblical text. At the same
time West realizes that Shechem's "sentiment expressed [was] probably rooted in sexual lust, rather than true love for Dinah."[58] This
scholar takes the part of the rapist because the Shechemites were
"friendly towards the invading Israelites and openly welcomed them."[59]
When read in relation to the rape, this statement is peculiar.

Nicolas Wyatt offers quite a different interpretation for the exalta-
tion of Shechem. Comparing Genesis 34 with ancient Near Eastern
texts, Wyatt classifies the biblical narrative as a relic of an archetypal
marriage rite similar to "the basic plot of premarital love" present in
Ugaritic and Akkadian texts.[60] To fit the comparison, Wyatt must
change the vocabulary of Genesis 34:2. He proposes to switch the
stem of ענה from the piel to the qal, so that the verb translates as "to
make love." This suggestion enables Wyatt to maintain that "the essence of the affair between Shechem and Dinah turns out to be substantially that of the other ancient near eastern forms."[61] He supports
his understanding of ענה with the following argument:

> A more innocent age than our own would have understood this as meaning
> simply that he spoke with her! Gen. 34.2 may therefore be understood simply
> as stating that Shechem made love to Dinah. We may even suppose that she
> was a willing partner, because far from possessing her out of selfish lust, we
> read immediately afterwards that he loved her and wanted to marry her.[62]

Aside from the question whether Shechem's love and marriage proposal
indicate Dinah's willingness, the words "more," "may," and "simply"

---

[55] Stuart A. West, "The Rape of Dinah and the Conquest of Shechem," *Dor le
Dor* 8, no. 3 (Spring 1980): 151f.

[56] Ibid., 148.

[57] Ibid., 145.

[58] Ibid., 148.

[59] Ibid., 152.

[60] Nicolas Wyatt, "The Story of Dinah and Shechem, " *Ugarit-Forschungen* 22
(1990): 434. His interpretation presupposes an original source as the basis for his
argument.

[61] Ibid., 436.

[62] Ibid.

exhibit the tentativeness of Wyatt's argument. In promoting it, Wyatt lays the groundwork for his main thesis that Genesis 34 reflects a sacred marriage ritual. Genesis 34 remains, however, unique in one respect. The account includes the "untimely death of one of the partners." And so Wyatt claims that the narrative "is hardly a tale of love requited and brought to fruition: it is *au contraire* a tale that ends in tragedy." Subordinating the biblical account to ancient Near Eastern texts, Wyatt reconstructs a story about a sacred marriage ritual. Unfortunately, in this version the bridegroom dies.

A Combination of Male Characters

A few scholars focus simultaneously on several of the male characters. Leon R. Kass chooses Jacob and his sons.[63] He claims that "only in this story can we see how the founders of Israel regard and treat a daughter" and "only in this story can we see how young Israelites regard and treat a sister."[64] Thus the father and brothers command his attention.

J. Gerald Janzen considers the brothers and Shechem "the primary actors."[65] He acknowledges the significance of Dinah's visit by asking, "What may happen when the women of the two societies get together?" He believes that "given the power-relations between the sexes, the rape is tragically no surprise." What Janzen finds "unexpected is Shechem's subsequent love for Dinah."[66] He sympathizes with Shechem when Shechem's "ruthless appetite . . . moderates into . . . the desire for marriage." By contrast, the brothers debase "the sacral institutions of marriage and circumcision . . . into weapons."[67] Janzen's conclusion is unclear. Integrating the story into the broader context of "the foundations of a new community through barren marriages that become fertile," he classifies Genesis 34 as "a study in the rape of justice." The rape of Dinah becomes a metaphor of "struggles for power

---

[63] Leon R. Kass, "Regarding Daughters and Sisters," *Commentary* 93, no. 4 (April 1992): 29. For the same focus see Nisan Ararat, "Reading According to the 'Seder' in the Biblical Narrative: To Balance the Reading of the Dinah Episode," *HaSifrut* 27 (December 1978): 15-34.

[64] Kass, "Regarding Daughters and Sisters," 30.

[65] J. Gerald Janzen, *Abraham and All the Families of the Earth: A Commentary on the Book of Genesis 12-50*, International Theological Commentary (Grand Rapids, MI: Eerdmans, 1993), 136.

[66] Ibid.

[67] Ibid., 137.

and wealth." By ending with a question, "That is to say, what will it take for the children of Jacob to become the children of Israel?,"[68] Janzen leaves the answer to the readers.

Victor P. Hamilton presents his interpretation in a verse-by-verse fashion that offers a multitude of details. Treating primarily the roles of the brothers and Shechem, he also states: "Throughout all of this violence and vendetta, not one word has been heard from Dinah."[69] Attempting to imagine her situation, Hamilton believes that "she is not the victim of impetuous and unbridled sexual impulses, to be discarded once sexual congress is completed. Shechem is romantically attracted to Dinah."[70] The focus turns to Shechem as her lover, though he also is the "villain."[71] Hamilton does not find a contradiction between these two descriptions. He understands rape as a "humbl[ing] or sham[ing]"[72] experience for Dinah. The title expresses this view: "The Humbling of Dinah,"[73] a euphemism that erases the accountability of the rapist. This understanding allows space for imagining Shechem to move from rape to love and to subsume "his violation" to his "passion."[74] Nevertheless, Hamilton characterizes Shechem as a "rogue"[75] because of his marriage proposal. This scholar applauds the brothers when they respond to the rape the first time: "They are indignant and beside themselves with rage, and rightly so."[76] However, the premise that "humbling" and "passion" are compatible enables Hamilton to refrain from condemning Shechem for the rape. Hamilton assumes that "maybe" the narrator depicts the brothers "as individuals of conscience and integrity."[77] He, however, hesitates to sympathize with them because he questions their attempt at "guarding Israel's purity at all cost."[78] The focus on the brothers and Shechem prevails, whether they are treated sympathetically or not.

---

[68] Ibid., 138.

[69] Victor P. Hamilton, *The Book of Genesis: Chapters 18-50*, New International Commentary on the Old Testament (Grand Rapids, MI: Eerdmans, 1995), 372.

[70] Ibid., 365.

[71] Ibid., 353.

[72] Ibid., 352.

[73] Ibid., 351.

[74] Ibid., 365.

[75] Ibid., 356.

[76] Ibid., 357.

[77] Ibid., 371.

[78] Ibid., 373.

George W. Coats also selected for attention the brothers, "princi-
pally Simeon and Levi," and Shechem along with his father Hamor.
The problem arises when "Shechem rapes Dinah but also loves her"
and wants "to convert the *strained* relationship into a permanent one"
[emphasis added].[79] The brothers oppose Shechem's "folly." Since the
rape merely "strains" the relationship between Shechem and Dinah,
the "simple plot [is] focused not on the rape of Dinah by Shechem, but
on the rape of Shechem by the brothers of Dinah." Consequently, the
title of this "simple plot" is "Rape of Shechem." The rapist is the
raped one and the rape of Dinah becomes an act of love. Not the rape
but "plunder leads to complication in the relationship between Israel
and Shechem." The brothers—and not Shechem—cause the "complication." Coats substantially transforms the biblical narrative.

Source Criticism

A number of scholars are not content to read Genesis 34 in its final
form. They detect sources within the text.[80] Recognizing the incom-
patibility of vv. 2 and 3, the juxtaposition of rape and "love,"[81] Samuel
Sandmel reasons that "two layers are found in the story, *for* the author of the later version was horrified at the implications of the basic
story" [stress added].[82] He claims that an earlier version reports the
love story of Shechem and Dinah: "Shechem fell in love with Dinah
and asked his father Hamor to arrange a marriage." Shechem accepts
the conditions of circumcision but the brothers nevertheless kill him
and the whole male community. This earlier version does not explain
why the brothers murdered the Shechemites. Making "significant al-
terations," the later version adds the rape to the story, the final fearful
response of Jacob, and the question of Simeon and Levi. The final
form represents the efforts of the later author who "was horrified at
the implications of the basic story." In his source critical approach,
Sandmel is wrestling with the ethical dilemmas of the narrative. De-

---

[79] This and the following quotes are from George W. Coats, *Genesis with an
Introduction to Narrative Literature*, The Forms of the Old Testament Literature,
ed. Rolf Knierim and Gene Tucker, vol. 1 (Grand Rapids, MI: Eerdmans, 1983), 234.

[80] For a concise summary see Paul Kevers, "Étude littéraire de Genése 34," *Revue Biblique* 87 (January 1980): 38-86.

[81] For an alternative translation of v. 3, see chapter 6.

[82] Samuel Sandmel, *The Hebrew Scriptures: An Introduction to Their Literature and Religious Ideas* (New York: Oxford University Press, 1978), 365.

spite this valiant effort to make sense of "a barbaric account," no formal elements support his positing of two layers.

Sandmel is not the only scholar who uses source criticism. Yair Zakovitch seeks "to reconstruct the original source"[83] in Genesis 34. He observes: "The sequence of actions at the beginning of the story is difficult: Shechem lay with the girl and ravished her (v. 2), and only afterward became infatuated with her and sought to persuade her (v. 3)."[84] Because of the anachronism in v. 7, the awkward syntax regarding the "defiling of Dinah" in vv. 13 and 27, and the "real tension over which of the brothers attacked the city of Shechem" in vv. 25-31, later editors added vv. 2b, 5, 7ab, 13a, 13b, 17, 25a, 25b, 27, 30, and 31.[85] The original story presented "Shechem's innocent attraction to Dinah and Jacob's sons' treacherous exploitation of the situation in order to plunder the city."[86] It did not contain "the rape element." Editors added the rape to supply a motive for the brothers.[87] They also assimilated the original story to two biblical texts: the story of the rape of Tamar (2 Samuel 13) and Jacob's curse of his two sons (Genesis 49:5-7). The assimilation of Genesis 34 to these texts results in a contrived story in which rape explains the fraternal violence.

Leslie Brisman holds that "a belated author had before him an ur-text corresponding to the work actually preserved in certain fragments of our present text."[88] Dividing Genesis 34 into two sources, he calls the "belated author" Jacob, and he "would like to call" the author of the non-Jacobic material "Eisaac" (Isaac). These sources do "not exactly" substitute for the sources commonly called "Jahwist" and "Elohist,"[89] but they are similar. The Eisaac version, the original literary source, did not contain the rape but told of Shechem's attraction to Dinah, his marriage proposal, and the "nationalistic" response of

---

[83] This and the following quotes are from Yair Zakovitch, "Assimilation in Biblical Narratives," in *Empirical Models for Biblical Criticism*, ed. Jeffrey H. Tigay (Philadelphia: University of Pennsylvania Press, 1985), 176.

[84] Ibid., 186.

[85] Ibid., 186f.

[86] Ibid., 188.

[87] Ibid., 189.

[88] Leslie Brisman, *The Voice of Jacob: On the Composition of Genesis* (Bloomington: Indiana University Press, 1990), xv. For another sympathetic focus on the J-source see Josef Scharbert, *Genesis 12-50* (Würzburg: Echter Verlag, 1986), 225-30.

[89] Brisman, *The Voice of Jacob*, xv.

the brothers. According to Brisman, "The Eisaacic story is a story not about rape but about the threat of assimilation."[90] Only the "Jacobic transformation of the Dinah story"[91] destroyed the positive image of Shechem. The Jacob source added the rape in v. 2, countered Shechem's "graciousness" in v. 4, and mocked it in v. 7 to "undermine the gentle pathos of Eisaac's story of Dinah." The Jacob source "quarrel[s]" with the Eisaac source. In this quarrel the former adds the rape to gain ground in "charges of moral right and wrong."[92] Throughout Brisman's interpretation the rape itself remains secondary.

Erhard Blum posits two sources. The original source stresses the innocence of Shechem and "the unreasonableness of the revenge of Simeon and Levi."[93] This source promotes a "pro-Shechemite version" which the later editor changes. In the earlier version, according to Blum, "the narrator does not get tired to stress the sincerity of Shechem's courtship for Dinah: v. 3 in the account of the narrator: his love for Dinah; v. 4: his intention to pay any bride price; v. 19 an interjection: Shechem's devotion to fulfill the condition."[94] Hence Blum insists that "it is beyond the question that *after* his deed Shechem meets his duty in *every* respect, since after all he desires to marry Dinah and he even agrees to pay an excessive bride price."[95] For Blum, the original narrator clearly denounces the brothers by juxtaposing Shechem's love to the fraternal vengenance. Only a later Judaic secondary tradition softened the image of the brothers.[96] Similar to other source critics, Blum construes an original love story that questions the proportion of the fraternal revenge to Shechem's "passion."

---

[90] Ibid., 92.

[91] Ibid., 95.

[92] Ibid., 96.

[93] Erhard Blum, *Die Komposition der Vätergeschichte* (Neukirchen-Vluyn: Neukirchener Verlag, 1984), 216: "die Unangemessenheit der Rache von Simeon und Levi." See also p. 213: "So scheint die Erzählung geradezu daraufhin angelegt zu sein, das ungerechtfertigte Übermaß der Rache von Simeon und Levi herauszustellen."

[94] Ibid., 211: "Der Erzähler wird nicht müde, die Aufrichtigkeit seiner Werbung um Dina hervorzuheben: V. 3 im Bericht des Erzählers: seine Liebe zu Dina; V. 4: seine Absicht, jeden Brautpreis zu bezahlen; V. 19 in einer Zwischenbemerkung: Sichems Eifer bei der Erfüllung der Bedingung."

[95] Ibid., 212: "steht es außer Frage, daß Sichem *nach* seiner Untat seiner Verpflichtung in jeder Hinsicht nachkommt, begehrt er doch Dina von sich aus zur Frau und ist sogar bereit, einen überhöhten Brautpreis zu bezahlen."

[96] Ibid., 229.

Unlike the preceding studies, Claus Westermann proposes three rather than two sources for Genesis 34. Source A was an original family or Shechem tradition, a "patriarchal story that tells of the revenge of two brothers for the outrage against their sister."[97] It contains the following verses: 1-3, 5-7, 11-12, 14, 25-26, 28, and 30-31. Source B, the tribal narrative or Hamor tradition, is "an account of the peaceful settlement of an Israelite group in the region of a Canaanite city."[98] It contains vv. 4, 6, 8-10, 13-17, 20-24a.b, 27-29, and 35:5. Source C is the final redaction. It draws upon Deuteronomy 7:1-5, a text prohibiting intermarriage and opposing the possibility of peaceful or contractual settlement. Further, it unites sources A and B to deliver a narrative that condemns intermarriage. Westermann postulates that source C changed "the account of the peaceful settlement of an Israelite group" in source B into a narrative of killing and plunder and integrated it with the "patriarchal story" of source A.

In arguing for three sources, Westermann does not focus on the rape. In fact, his reconstruction of source A combines the report about the rape (v. 2) with the report of Shechem's "love" (v. 3) without acknowledging the tension between them. According to Westermann, the "forceful violation" (v. 2) and Shechem's "speaking feelingly"[99] (v. 3) present a coherent narrative about Shechem.

Tribal History

In several studies Genesis 34 is read as a reflection of the early tribal history in ancient Israel. Michael Maher claims: "It is very probable that the story echoes the memory of a time when Simeon and Levi were quite powerful tribes" because "the idea that two men could slaughter all the males in the city . . . is rather far-fetched and indicates that we should not take the story literally."[100] Maher refers to

[97] Claus Westermann, *Genesis 12-36: A Commentary*, trans. J. J. Scullion (Minneapolis: Augsburg, 1985), 537. For an abbreviated version of the same argument see Claus Westermann, *Genesis: A Practical Commentary*, trans. David E. Green (Grand Rapids, MI: Eerdmans, 1987), 235-41.

[98] Westermann, *Genesis 12-36*, 536-37.

[99] Ibid., 538. The compatibility of vv. 2 and 3 is also supported by Stephen Mitchell, *Genesis: A New Translation of the Classic Biblical Stories* (New York: HarperCollins, 1996), 72-73.

[100] Michael Maher, *Genesis* (Wilmington: Glazier, 1982), 196. For a comprehensive study of the city of Shechem and the relationship of Israelite tribes to the city with reference to Genesis 34 see Eckart Otto, *Jakob in Sichem: Überlieferungsgeschichtliche, archäologische und territorialgeschichtliche Studien zur Entstehungsgeschichte Israels* (Stuttgart: Kohlhammer Verlag, 1979), esp. 169-81.

"modern commentators" in general who "believe that there is more to
this curious narrative than the story of individuals who got caught up
in the unfortunate consequences of a young man's amorous folly."[101]
The rape disappears behind the theory of early Israelite tribal settlement.

K. Luke discusses Genesis 34 as "a piece of tribal history."[102] The
narrative emerges as "an ethnological saga . . . a bitter and bloody
conflict" between the Shechemites and the tribes of Simeon and Levi
before 1200 B.C.E.[103] Aside from the fact that recent biblical scholarship has questioned the possibility of such early dating,[104] Luke's historical reconstruction of the tribal conflict does not include the rape.
One reason for this omission might be Luke's understanding of the
crime. Rather than finding rape, he turns to sexual perversion and
sacred prostitution:

> The reason why the Israelites attributed a crime of sexual perversion to the
> Shechemites is not a problem at all, for . . . the Canaanites were engaged in
> such practices as sacred prostitution, etc. which were abominations in the
> eyes of the people of Israel.[105]

This dismissal appears also in Luke's treatment of the individual
characters. They personify the tribes which Luke nevertheless interprets individually. Blaming Dinah for the rape, Luke writes that her
"feminine curiosity" caused the "trouble." The interpreter excuses the
rapist because "no doubt" Shechem liked Dinah and attempted to marry
her.[106] Shechem "abducted and violated her" since he "took a *fancy*
for the nomad girl"[107] [stress added]. Although Luke mentions the rape,
the word "fancy" neutralizes it. Counting the whole chapter "as a

---

[101] Maher, *Genesis*, 196.

[102] K. Luke, *Studies on the Book of Genesis* (Alwaye, India: Assisi Press, 1975),
126. For a brief reference to Genesis 34 as part of the tribal history see Richard J.
Clifford and Roland E. Murphy, "Genesis," in *The New Jerome Biblical Commentary*, ed. Raymond E. Brown, Joseph A. Fitzmyer, and Roland E. Murphy (Englewood
Cliffs, NJ: Prentice-Hall, 1990), 34-35.

[103] Luke, *Genesis,* 133.

[104] See Philip R. Davies, *In Search of 'Ancient Israel'* (Sheffield, UK: JSOT
Press, 1992); Keith Whitelam, *The Invention of Ancient Israel: The Silencing of
Palestinian History* (London: Routledge, 1996).

[105] Luke, *Genesis,* 134.

[106] Ibid., 128.

[107] Luke, *Genesis*, 127.

[108] Ibid., 126.

piece of the tribal history,"[108] Luke aims to accentuate "God's lordship over history."[109]

Luke is not alone in using tribal history to evade the topic of rape. For Nahum M. Sarna "the characters of the story are really personifications, corporate personalities," so that "Gen. 34 records an incident that belongs to the prehistory of the Israelite tribes."[110] His evaluation includes neither an explanation of the rape as part of the tribal confrontation nor a characterization of Dinah as the personification of a tribe.

These issues emerge in the tribal interpretation of Robert Davidson. Going back "beyond the present personalized form,"[111] Davidson understands Genesis 34 as "some incident during the settlement of some Hebrew group or groups in Canaan." Although Davidson acknowledges Genesis 34 as "the only story which tradition has preserved concerning Dinah, the daughter of Jacob," the "historical kernel" of the story concerns "a violent seizure of Shechem." This "old story" describes a conflict between the city of Shechem, "an important Canaanite communication centre in the central highlands," and the tribal groups of Israel. The rape does not feature in it.

The literary study of Paul Kevers also claims that Genesis 34 describes the relations between different population groups as exemplified by individual characters. Whereas Shechem and the two brothers are the main representatives of ancient clans, Dinah and Jacob remain marginal. For Kevers the narrative describes the conflict of different ethnic Israelite tribes that disagree about intermarriage. The rape qua rape becomes irrelevant.[112]

The famous Genesis commentary of Gerhard von Rad made a significant contribution to interpreting chapter 34 as a part of tribal history. Revising his commentary only months before his death, von Rad

---

[109] Ibid., 136.

[110] Nahum M. Sarna, "The Ravishing of Dinah: A Commentary on Genesis 34," in *Studies in Jewish Education and Judaica in Honor of Louis Newman*, ed. Alexander M. Shapiro and Burton I. Cohen (New York: Ktav, 1984), 155. For a similar view see Jan Dus, *Israelitische Vorfahren—Vasallen palästinischer Stadtstaaten? Revisionsbedürftigkeit der Landnahmehypothese von Albrecht Alt*, European University Studies 23, vol. 404 (Frankfurt: Lang, 1991).

[111] This and the following quotes are from Robert Davidson, *Genesis 12-50*, Cambridge Bible Commentary (Cambridge, UK: Cambridge University Press, 1979), 194.

[112] Kevers, "Étude littéraire," 72ff.

wrote: "The narrative seems to go back to the time when Israelite tribes were not yet settled in Palestine but on their way thither in search of new pasture."[113] He continues:

> By some catastrophe they were pushed out of the territory around Shechem and other tribes could settle there later. The essential intention of the narrative in its present form is to present this prehistoric conflict of Simeon and Levi. But like many sagas it has changed the political proceedings into a conflict of fewer single persons and accordingly illustrated it on the level of the personal and universally human.

In this reconstruction of tribal history the rape becomes an unspecified "catastrophe." Even though von Rad entitles the section "The Rape of Dinah," his concluding remarks do not even mention it. One reason might be that in the personalized version of the "saga" Shechem "has fallen in love with the girl, Dinah." The brothers of Dinah, Simeon and Levi, "seek to purify the honor of their violated sister at the cost of a morally ambiguous deed." Again, love is heralded, and the brothers turn into morally ambiguous characters. Although von Rad acknowledges the rape on the level of the personal, he values Shechem and his love. "The emphasis on the great love for the girl, which brooks no hindrance, receives the benefit of the narrative, and the figure of Shechem is made more human for the reader."[114] Overall, however, the particular features of the narrative disappear for the sake of larger historical considerations that place Genesis 34 within Israelite tribal history.

Interpreting the final verse (v. 31), the open-ended question of the brothers to their father, von Rad provides perhaps a reason for his preference:

> And the ancient reader, who *felt more than we do* the burning shame done to the brothers in the rape of Dinah, will not have called them wrong. [stress added][115]

Apparently, von Rad does not sympathize with the brothers and Dinah because he seems to feel little of "the burning shame" the brothers felt for their sister. Of course, von Rad presupposes that the broth-

---

[113] This and the following quotes are from Gerhard von Rad, *Genesis: A Commentary*, 3d rev. ed. (Philadelphia: Westminster Press, 1972), 329.

[114] Ibid., 331.

[115] Ibid., 334.

ers felt "shame." The narrator, however, never describes their feelings as shame (בוש) but instead as sadness (יתעצב) and depression (יחר ל). Lacking empathy for Dinah, von Rad favors Shechem's "love."

Xenophobia

An Anthropological Approach

Some scholars regard the issue of xenophobia as the interpretive focus of Genesis 34. They maintain that fear of the Canaanite neighbors motivates a narrative which struggles between integration and exclusion. One of those proposing such an interpretation is Lyn M. Bechtel. She suggests that Genesis 34 reflects the dispute within Israel. As a group-oriented society, Israel was divided as to whether to interact with non-Israelites and to cross tribal boundaries or not.[116] The characters represent the different positions. One faction—personified by Dinah and Jacob—wants to interact with outsiders. The other groups—personified by the brothers, "the militant folks"—votes for separation and group "purity." Bechtel believes the writers of Genesis 34 oppose the excluding position: "The story seems to be challenging this attitude [of the brothers] by showing the potential danger in which it places the group."[117]

Relying on anthropology, Bechtel explains that individuals lived and worked to serve the good of the larger group. In such a society the differentiation between "us" and "them" was essential. "Closely knit" boundaries had to be maintained. The activities of individuals strengthened the boundaries. Marriage was a group affair and sexual intercourse perpetuated the values of the family and clan. Sexual intercourse became shameful only when it lacked family or community bonding. Dinah and Shechem, however, are "two unbonded people"[118] when they have "intercourse." The question therefore is not whether rape occurred but whether the "sexual intercourse" between Shechem and Dinah was shameful.

---

[116] Lyn M. Bechtel, "What If Dinah Is Not Raped? (Genesis 34)," *Journal for the Study of the Old Testament* 62 (June 1994): 19-36. A similar focus is proposed by Bernd Jörg Diebner, "Gen 34 und Dinas Rolle bei der Definition 'Israels,'" *Dielheimer Blätter zum Alten Testament* 19 (July 1984): 59-75. Diebner reconstructs the controversy from the perspective of "Jerusalem's orthodoxy" during the second century B.C.E.

[117] Bechtel, "What If Dinah", 36.

[118] Ibid., 27.

Referring to texts like Deuteronomy 22:23-29, Bechtel shows that Deuteronomic law considered sexual intercourse as shameful only when it threatened the social bonding of the community. Shechem, however, does not threaten the social bonding of the community. He tries to win approval from the other group, proposes marriage and offers many goods. His father, Hamor, supports him. "The text stresses that these are honorable men" and that "the overall action of Shechem . . . is one of honor." And so she concludes: "Throughout the text there is no indication that Dinah is raped. The description of Shechem's behavior and attitude does not fit that of a rapist."[119] Consequently, "all of this diminishes the likelihood that rape was seen to have occurred."[120]

In addition, Bechtel claims that biblical Hebrew does not have a specific term for rape. Instead, the verb ענה "reflects the process of status manipulation inherent in shaming." It indicates "humiliation or shaming of a woman through certain kinds of sexual intercourse including rape, though not necessarily."[121] In Genesis 34, however, the intercourse is not shameful because Shechem proposes to marry Dinah.

Excusing Shechem, Bechel considers the brothers as the villains. Stuck in an exclusionary group-oriented behavior that threatens to destroy the wider community, the brothers retreat to unjustifiable vengeance which is later condemned (Genesis 49:5-7). According to Bechtel, the brothers manifest their inferiority through cunning and do not see that "in the long run this kind of behavior violates group-oriented ideals. . . ." Echoing scholars who use hermeneutical approaches, Bechtel says: "Ironically, if there is a rape in this story, it is Simeon and Levi who 'rape' the Shechemites."[122] Again, the killing turns to rape and the rape into acceptable intercourse.

---

[119] Ibid., 31. Cf. also Carolyn Pressler, "Sexual Violence and Deuteronomic Law," in *A Feminist Companion to Exodus and Deuteronomy* (Sheffield: Sheffield University Press, 1994), 111, who argues similarly: "For example, the Deuteronomic laws suggest that the question of whether Shechem raped or seduced Dinah (Gen. 34) is moot. If the same assumptions are operating in the Deuteronomic laws and in the Dinah story, then the offense in the story is not that Shechem had sexual intercourse with Dinah without her consent. It is that Shechem had sexual intercourse with Dinah without her father's or brothers' consent."

[120] Bechtel, "What If Dinah", 29. Cf. also Tikva Frymer-Kensky, "The Law and Philosophy: The Case of Sex in the Bible," *Semeia* 45 (1989): 89-102, esp. 95.

[121] Ibid., 24.

[122] Ibid., 34.

Bechtel's extensive discussion merits a number of criticisms, the first being that the study relies entirely on the anthropological concept of group-oriented societies without explicitly discussing anthropological literature. In footnote 5 Bechtel refers to one study published in 1967. The examination of more recent anthropolical studies might have stimulated a discussion about the problems involved when scholars transfer concepts developed in twentieth-century scholarship to ancient Israel. Anthropologist John K. Chance voiced such a concern in a response to studies which relied on the anthropological concept of "honor and shame" in the Bible. He cautions biblical scholars not to "upstream," that is "to project insights gained in the twentieth century . . . back into the distant past."[123]

A second criticism is that Bechtel authorizes her translation of ענה as "to humiliate" incorrectly with the dictionary of W. Baumgartner. The dictionary translates the piel of the verb in Genesis 34:2 as "to commit a rape (on a woman) Genesis 34:2"[124] and underlines that the piel indicates "to do violence to someone." Although Bechtel refers to the dictionary, her interpretation does not mention this emphasis.[125]

Third, Bechtel criticizes biblical scholars for "automatically" assuming that Shechem raped Dinah.[126] Her critique, however, does not consider that numerous scholars interpreted Genesis 34 as a love story between Dinah and Shechem, as a story of seduction and an attempted marriage, destroyed by the brothers. Bechtel's study is another example of what has already been examined in chapter 3 and in this chapter—the various ways scholars read Genesis 34 not as a narrative about rape. Furthermore, a footnote about "some feminists [for whom] the story becomes a paradigm of many situations of rape in modern society"[127] could have provided more specific information of such attempts and not only dismissed them.

Fourth, Bechtel suggests that the verb ענה in the piel should be translated as "to shame, humiliate." She, however, does not explain two other texts that are usually accepted as references to rape: Judges

[123] John K. Chance, "The Anthropology of Honor and Shame: Culture, Values, and Practice," *Semeia: Honor and Shame in the World of the Bible* 68 (1996): 141.

[124] Ludwig Köhler and Walter Baumgartner, eds., *Lexicon in Veteris Testamenti Libros* (Leiden/Grand Rapids, MI: Brill/Eerdmans, 1958), 719.

[125] Bechtel, "What if Dinah," 23-24.

[126] Ibid., 19.

[127] Ibid., 20.

19:24 and Lamentations 5:11. The *New Revised Standard Version* (NRSV) translates them, "They wantonly raped her" (Judges 19:24) and, "Women are raped in Zion" (Lamentations 5:11). Since Bechtel proposes that the verb does not mean "to rape," in her view the two verses might not refer to rape either.

The fifth and final criticism of Bechtel's refers to her emphasis on the Deuteronomic law for interpreting Genesis 34. Bechtel presupposes that the legal code preceded the narrative. Other scholars suggest the opposite order. For example, Calum M. Carmichael claims that Genesis 34 preceded the Deuteronomic laws.[128] In his view the narrative serves as the basis for developing the legal code. One might also assume that the Deuteronomist developed the laws according to changed circumstances, so that the legal codes did not relate to the narrative. It seems that whatever the connection between the two, no definite order can be assumed.

Collage Interpretations

Walter Brueggemann similarly promotes Genesis 34 as a discussion on xenophobia. For him, the theme is "Israelite accommodation to non-Israelites in the land . . . a much disputed issue in Israel."[129] And so "the liaison of Dinah and Shechem" refers to the interaction between Canaanites and Israelites which Brueggemann considers to be the result of a "seduction." Israel, however, considers intermarriage as "perversion." Therefore, "the report on Shechem is obviously given from a polemical Israelite perspective."[130] Judging the brothers, Brueggemann states that "this narrative evidences the unsophisticated and irrational response of a passion unencumbered by reflection."[131] The brothers are not interested in "accommodation, cooperation, or

---

[128] Carmichael, *Women, Law, and the Genesis Traditions*, passim.

[129] Walter Brueggemann, *Genesis: A Bible Commentary for Teaching and Preaching* (Atlanta: Knox Press, 1982), 274. See also Johanna Hooysma, "Die Vergewaltigung Dinas: Auslegung von Gen. 33, 18-34, 31," *Texte & Kontexte* 30 (July 1986): 26-46, who reads Genesis 34 as a debate about mixed marriages in postexilic Judah. Lothar Ruppert, *Das Buch Genesis*, Teil II: *Kap. 25, 19-50, 26*, Geistliche Schriftlesung 6/2 (Düsseldorf: Patmos Verlag, 1984), sees in it a reference to Israelite and Canaanite contact. Shechem receives sympathy for his "true" love (p. 144). The brothers, however, receive "God's mercy," like Ruppert's fellow Christians (p. 155). For a focus on xenophobia see also Moshe Weinfeld, *The Book of Genesis*, Encyclopedia of the World of the Tanakh (Rabibim, 1982).

[130] Brueggeman, *Genesis*, 275.

[131] Ibid., 276.

even ratification." Vengeance dominates them.[132] "Fixed on the narrow sexual issue," they are "blind to the larger economic issues, blind to the dangers they have created, blind to the possibilities of cooperation, and blind even to the ways they have compromised their own religion in their thirst for vengeance and gain." Understandably for Brueggemann, Jacob despairs over his sons. The father's attempt to achieve a "more pragmatic settlement" with Shechem makes more sense to Brueggemann than the fraternal response. Jacob, however, could not prevail against the "more sectarian and destructive settlement" of his sons.[133] Lacking "social cooperation," "ecumenical community," and "economic advantage,"[134] the brothers do not elicit sympathy from Brueggemann who wishes them "faith" to release their "resolution of passion."[135]

The brief interpretation of William H. Propp also condemns the reaction of the brothers. In his view, as a story about the relationship between the Israelites and Canaanites, Genesis 34 "is not a record of assimilation but a reaction to it presenting various attitudes with the voices of the protagonists."[136] One group favors intermarriage; another opposes it. In Propp's analysis, even the Canaanites could be the authors of Genesis 34; they could have created the narrative "as a pretext for avoiding marriage with the Israelites."[137] Another possibility would be an Israelite author who "seems most sympathetic to the accommodationists," that is, Jacob and the Shechemites. In this speculation about the "accommodationists" the issue of rape disappears.

Seth Daniel Kunin regards Genesis 34 as an expression of the struggle involving the "amalgamation of peoples," which the narrative opposes on both the individual and the national level: "The text implies that Dinah improperly joined the Canaanite women and thus

---

[132] Ibid., 278.

[133] Ibid., 279.

[134] Ibid., 278.

[135] Ibid., 279.

[136] William H. Propp, "The Origins of Infant Circumcision in Israel," *Hebrew Annual Review* 11 (1987): 355-70. For a similar argument proposed for a later setting see J. A. Soggin, "Genesis Kapitel 34. Eros und Thanatos," in *History and Traditions of Early Israel*, ed. André Lemaire and Benedikt Otzen, Supplements to Vetus Testamentum 50 (Leiden: Brill, 1993), 133-35. See Wilhelm Th. in der Smitten, "Gen 34—Ausdruck der Volksmeinung," *Bibliotheca Orientalis* 30, no. 1-2 (1973): 7-9.

[137] Propp, "The Origins of Infant Circumcision," 360f.

created the situation of danger."[138] The adverb "improperly" does not appear in Genesis 34. By adding it, Kunin blames Dinah for the rape. Unfortunately, he misidentifies the rapist by calling him Hamor rather than Shechem.[139]

Terry J. Prewitt presents an intriguing twist. He compares Genesis 34 not with other rape narratives but with marriage stories that are disruptive or supportive of "patrilineage" in ancient Israel.[140] Such stories include the marriage of Abraham and Sarah, Isaac and Rebekah, Jacob, Leah, and Rachel, and even Joseph.[141] Prewitt also compares Genesis 34 with "redemption narratives" which "introduce cultural themes limiting or defining appropriate action of members of immediate households."[142] One of the charts Prewitt provides proposes that the marriage of Dinah to Shechem would have been redemptive if the xenophobia of the brothers had not prevented the "redemption."[143] He writes: "When Simeon and Levi kill Shechem, they eliminate Dinah's husband."[144] Further, they prevent the application of the Levirate rule (Deuteronomy 25:5-10) by killing not only Shechem but every male in the town. Thus, the writers of the book of Genesis stress that "genealogical distance produces [a] greater probability of distrust among agnatic kinsmen."[145] The authors use chapter 34 to "reassert the idea that the transformation of a distant agnate or rank-equivalent male into an in-law, an ally by marriage, maintains social cohesion and political strength."[146] The brothers misunderstand the advantages of such a marriage. Read as a "false or unsuccessful marriage offer,"[147] Genesis 34 illustrates the xenophobia of the brothers. For Prewitt, rape is not the issue.

---

[138] Seth Daniel Kunin, *The Logic of Incest: A Structuralist Analysis of Hebrew Mythology* (Sheffield, UK: Sheffield Academic Press, 1995), 137.

[139] Ibid., 138. The incorrect name of the rapist appears also in footnote 1 on the same page.

[140] Terry J. Prewitt, *The Elusive Covenant: A Structural-Semiotic Reading of Genesis* (Bloomington: Indiana University Press, 1990), 100.

[141] Ibid., 98.

[142] Ibid., 107.

[143] Ibid., 108.

[144] Ibid., 109.

[145] Ibid., 106. See also the chart on p. 86, which classifies Genesis 34 as a "false or unsuccessful marriage offer, breach of marriage by women."

[146] Ibid., 107.

[147] Ibid., 86.

A similar approach appears in the recent historical speculations of Hartmut N. Rösel. Focusing on the relation of Israel and Canaan in the book of Genesis, Rösel says: "It is clear that the narrative of Genesis 34 is dominated by the problem of living together between the Israelite and non-Israelite population."[148] As a representative of the Canaanites, Shechem offends "a sexual taboo of Israel" by "lying" with Dinah and only afterward seeking marriage, the reversal of "the usual succession."[149] In this interpretation premarital sex is the problem because Shechem disregards the custom of marrying the woman before having sex with her. Nevertheless, his offer to marry her is a commendable act, according to Rösel. As representatives of "Israelite circles," the brothers reject the "respectable" behavior of Shechem and a peaceful life with the Canaanites. Along with other biblical stories this one testifies to the Israelite need to accept the Canaanite population. The process ranges from assimilation to violent conflicts. Genesis 34 propagates the latter. It is an anti-Canaanite solution.

Recently, Ralph W. Klein argues a similar point. Exploring the theme of globalization, he reviews "three occasions when Israel's life intersected with that of its neighbors, and when its response to these 'others' was characterized by ambivalence and ambiguity and by courageous hope that would not settle for the status quo."[150] "The Case of Dinah" is one such occasion.

Before Klein shows how Genesis 34 relates to the issue of globalization, he acknowledges the following: "A majority of commentators believe" that the foreigner Shechem raped Dinah.[151] Read this way,

---

[148] Hartmut N. Rösel, *Israel in Kanaan: Zum Problem der Entstehung Israels*, Beiträge zur Erforschung des Alten Testaments und des Antiken Judentums 11 (Frankfurt: Lang, 1992), 41: "Es ist deutlich, daß die Erzählung Gen 34 von der Problematik des Zusammenlebens von israelitischer und nichtisraelitischer Bevölkerung geprägt ist." For a similar evaluation see Jairah Amit, "A Hidden Polemic in the Story of the Rape of Dinah (Hebrew)," in *Proceedings of the Eleventh World Congress of Jewish Studies, Division A: The Bible and Its World*, ed. David Assaf (Jerusalem: Magnes Press, 1994), 1-8. Amit, however, dates Genesis 34 toward the end of the Second Temple Period as a "hidden" polemic against marriage with the Samaritans. For a description of his method in English see Jairah Amit, "Hidden Polemic in the Conquest of Dan: Judges 17-18," *Vetus Testamentum* 60 (1990): 4-20.

[149] Rösel, *Israel in Kanaan*, 40.

[150] Ralph W. Klein, "Israel/Today's Believers and the Nations: Three Test Cases," *Currents in Theology and Mission* 24, no. 3 (June 1997): 232.

[151] Ibid., 233.

Dinah emerges as "a classic victim of rape or even date rape" and "Shechem seems to be the completely abusive male, having his own way sexually and then professing his love and many 'sweet nothings' to the one he has violated (v. 3)."[152] Considering this scenario, Klein recommends: "We all do well to be angry about this incident." Klein's unequivocal rejection of the rapist and his anger about the rape is both rare and a much-needed correction in the history of interpretation.

However, Klein's interest in Genesis 34 arises from a different concern. He proposes "an alternative interpretation" in which the issue is not the rape but "whether we the readers are ready to be open to the 'other'." This understanding requires a modification for v. 2, and so Klein admits: "The crux of this interpretation rests in the translation of v. 2." Like other scholars, Klein maintains that "no one denies that Shechem 'took her' and 'lay with her', but the NRSV's addition of 'by force' may miss the whole point. What was controversial about the sexual liaison of Shechem and Dinah is that it brought shame or defilement on Dinah, at least in the view of some of the characters in the story, because it was a relationship that crossed ethnic boundaries." The problem culminates in v. 31 where an open-ended question places the dilemma of crossing ethnic boundaries or not into the readers' laps. According to Klein, the narrator did not intend to resolve the issue but forced "all subsequent readers to debate, to rethink the implications of the faith, and then to make a choice."[153]

Interested in enriching the discussion about foreigners with biblical stories, Klein recommends Dinah as the model for contemporary readers. As she goes out to visit the women of the region, so contemporary readers could learn that "God's greatest gift is the transcendence of all cultural, ethnic, political and religious boundaries."[154] This discussion of xenophobia attributes a central role to Dinah. However, the significance of v. 2 is dismissed.

Feminist Approaches

In recent years several commentators have identified their interpretations of Genesis 34 as "feminist." They are examined in this section because the various scholars all name their readings feminist. However, in some cases their methodology and approach could also be

---

[152] This and the following quotes are from ibid., 234.
[153] Ibid., 235.
[154] Ibid., 237.

compared to emphases described above. Four categories describe the different feminist foci.

Work of Redaction

Reading from a feminist perspective,[155] Ita Sheres analyzes the connection between the redactors and Dinah to show how their "unfavorable attitude to women" shaped their edition of the narrative. She compares Dinah to the biblical women Eve, Rebekah, and Rachel and relates Genesis 34 to the contemporary Israeli situation. The perspective of the redactors is so important because "it was the redactors who put the final stamp on the portrait of Dinah as well as on those of all the other men and women in the text; and the specific manner in which Dinah appears in the text is due mainly to their ideological convictions."[156] The descripton of these convictions is a goal in this reading.

The attempt to establish the intentionality of the author or redactors is fraught with problems. According to Ricoeur, "the author's intention is beyond our reach,"[157] so that "understanding has less than ever to do with the author and his [sic] situation."[158] The reader brings a mute text to life. Hence, Sheres discloses her views when she reconstructs the intention of the redactors. When she writes that "Dinah was portrayed first of all as a victim; but she was also a responsible party in the crime because she undertook the forbidden [by the redactors] act of 'going out to see the women of the land,' "[159] Sheres assigns an opinion to the assumed redactors and thus presents her view.

---

[155] Ita Sheres, *Dinah's Rebellion: A Biblical Parable for Our Time* (New York: Crossroad, 1990), 114. In the foreword to the book (p. vii) David Noel Freedman also claims that Sheres writes from a feminist perspective. With a focus on biblical women, Jon L. Berquist wrote *Reclaiming Her Story: The Witness of Women in the Old Testament* (St. Louis: Chalice Press, 1992), which includes several pages on Dinah (pp. 61-65). Berquist does not label his interpretation "feminist." Thus, his work is not included in the following analysis. It should be noted that he blames the text for blaming Dinah for the rape, condemns the brothers, and believes in Shechem's "true love" (p. 62).

[156] Sheres, *Dinah's Rebellion*, 3.

[157] See Paul Ricoeur, *Interpretation Theory* (Fort Worth: Texas Christian University Press, 1976), 75. For a brief introduction to the history of intentionality in literary criticism see Annabel Patterson, "Intention," in *Critical Terms for Literary Study*, ed. Frank Lentricchia and Thomas McLaughlin (Chicago: University of Chicago Press, 1990), 135-46.

[158] Ricoeur, *Interpretation*, 87.

[159] Sheres, *Dinah's Rebellion*, 8.

Although the text does not classify Dinah's visit as forbidden, Sheres describes the redactors' opinion about Dinah's behavior with this adjective. When she writes several pages later that Dinah's "rape is portrayed both as the result of her *unthoughtful* behavior and as an *instant* punishment for disobeying the rules spelled out by the men of the tribe" [stress added],[160] it is again Sheres who judges. The passive construction of the sentence and the adjectives do not derive from an "essentially male orientation" of the text but from Sheres herself.[161] Although she intends only to repeat the bad news, she, in fact, creates it.

Another example illustrates the problem of Sheres' interpretation. In the appendix Sheres reconstructs the story of Dinah "in its unredacted, reconstructed state."[162] This original form of the story does not contain the rape, "since structurally and linguistically it is difficult to accept his 'rape' of Dinah."[163] Similarly, the "bloody confrontation" between the Shechemites and the tribe of Simeon and Levi belongs to another source. Sheres hypothesizes that in the original story the heroine Dinah goes out to seek a husband, finds him in Shechem, and becomes his legitimate wife. Based on the original story, the final edition contains the elements that portray Shechem sympathetically. And so Sheres claims that "Shechem is the only person in the tale that is sympathetic to Dinah." He is depicted as "a man in love."[164]

> If one is to find male compassion in the story, one has to turn to Shechem, "the stranger," who after the rape falls in love with Dinah and realizes that he must "console the girl" before proceeding with official, ritualized courtship. Excluding all the other difficulties that this peculiar order of events suggests, it is fair to observe (as the text *unambiguously* does) that the only man sympathetic to Dinah is Shechem, the presumed villain of the piece. In fact, it can be easily argued that Shechem's attitude is not only the *most human* but also the *most credible*: how else could he have expected to live with Dinah, whom he had raped, as his wife?[165] [stress added]

---

[160] Ibid., 17.
[161] Ibid., 33.
[162] Ibid., 18, an early reference to the appendix on pp. 130-39.
[163] Ibid., 136.
[164] Ibid., 137.
[165] Ibid., 111f. For another critique of this view see Judith S. Antonelli, *In the Image of God: A Feminist Commentary on the Torah* (Northvale, NJ: Jason Aronson, 1996), 93-94.

Sheres sympathizes with the rapist and finds him the "most human" and the "most credible" character. Shechem is the hero because he "loves Dinah, and there is no indication that the attraction is not mutual."[166]

In writing about the women of Genesis, Sharon Pace Jeansonne attempts to discover the meaning of the redactor whom she calls narrator. Although she does not explicitly call her reading "feminist," she refers to the "patriarchal bias" of modern interpreters and "the advent of feminist hermeneutics."[167] Interested in the "relevance of the women within the ancestral history of Israel,"[168] she wonders where the reader's "sentiments"[169] should lie when the story ends. This question leads her to emphasize the "unresolved ambiguities."[170] On the one hand, "Dinah was only visiting the *women* of the land—she was not trying to put herself in any position to encounter the men of the land or to marry a Canaanite."[171] Her activity does not deserve rape because Dinah visits "only" the women. On the other hand, Shechem's love redeems the rape, so that the fraternal revenge is too harsh. Jeansonne also tries to redeem Dinah by downplaying the significance of those whom Dinah visited. In the end, however, Jeansonne focuses on the narrator, who shows "us many aspects of this crime and its repercussions."[172] Ambiguity prevails.

Role of Brothers
Ilona N. Rashkow presents a short analysis from a "feminist-psychological approach" in which she accuses the brothers of subjugating "female desire to male rule." Characterizing not the rape but the fraternal question in v. 31, "Should our sister be treated like a whore?" (NRSV), as the quintessential expression of male dominance, Rashkow

---

[166] Sheres, *Dinah's Rebellion*, 105. In the interpretation of Christine Friebe-Baron, *Ferne Schwestern, ihr seid mir nah: Begegnungen mit Frauen aus biblischer Zeit* (Stuttgart: Kreuz Verlag, 1988), 52-58, Shechem's love overrules the rape: "Aber immerhin war seine Leidenschaft dir zugewandt . . . ." (p. 55).

[167] Sharon Pace Jeansonne, *The Women of Genesis: From Sarah to Potiphar's Wife* (Minneapolis: Fortress, 1990), 1, 2.

[168] Ibid., 2.

[169] Ibid., 88.

[170] Ibid., 97.

[171] Ibid., 91.

[172] Ibid., 97.

states that the brothers "really castrated" Dinah.[173] Describing them
as "suddenly obsessed with a sense of outraged personal honor,"[174]
Rashkow believes that the brothers destroyed the opportunity for Dinah
to marry Shechem and live a respectful life with him.

Susan Niditch also emphasizes the role of the brothers. The issue is
not Dinah, who "recedes into the background."[175] It is "woman-steal-
ing and male honor." Shechem "helped himself to Dinah's sexuality,"[176]
is Niditch's way of describing the rape. She claims that the story contrasts male groups seeking to "repossess the woman." Fraternal trickery is the kernel of the narrative. "Streetsmart," the trickster warriors
use deception to protect their sister and get her back. Although Niditch
does not explicitly censure the brothers, she tells us from her "feminist
perspective"[177] that "the trickster ideology of war has the potential to
produce unabashedly and uncontrolledly violent behavior."[178] This ideology appeals "most to those outside the power structure."[179]

The Metaphor of Rape

Alice A. Keefe proposes that in Genesis 34 a "woman's experience
become[s] a signifier for broader issues of community."[180] She correlates rape to war to understand the biblical connection of sexuality
and violence. Not "women's sexuality" but rape as "the *violation* of
female sexuality" [stress added][181] is disruptive. Keefe claims that this
rape becomes "a metaphorical way of speaking" about the hostility
between Israelites and Canaanites. The narrative is "a way of speaking of its [Israel's] struggle to retain a distinctive and separate cultural
identity." The rape "serves as an expression of Israel's vulnerability to
being dominated, taken over and absorbed by the other peoples, par-

---

[173] Ilona N. Rashkow, *The Phallacy of Genesis: A Feminist-Psychological Approach* (Louisville, KY: Westminster and Knox Press, 1993), 106.

[174] Ibid., 105.

[175] Susan Niditch, *War in the Hebrew Bible: A Study in the Ethics of Violence*
(New York: Oxford University Press, 1993), 110.

[176] Ibid., 109.

[177] Ibid., 107.

[178] Ibid., 113.

[179] Ibid., 119.

[180] Alice A. Keefe, "Rapes of Women/Wars of Men," *Semeia* 61 (1993): 80. For
a brief interpretation focused on the rape and written by laypeople see Rose Sallberg
Kam, *Their Stories, Our Stories: Women of the Bible* (New York: Continuum,
1995), 66-71. Kam understands rape as an *individual* atrocity for "women."

[181] Keefe, "Rapes of Women," 82.

ticularly by urban Canaanite culture."[182] Dinah is then a metaphoric character through whom Israel imagines itself as a violated woman.

For Keefe, the story exemplifies the Israelite phenomenon to express "cultural encounter" at "the site of sexuality." "The female body functions as both a literal medium of exchange between peoples and a symbolic locus of 'intercourse' or encounter."[183] Through the violation of the woman's body Israel learns to see its social chaos. Keefe maintains that "woman's body [becomes] a sign for community, connectedness, and covenant . . . through images of victimization and violation. . . ."[184] Israelite writers created this rape narrative to fight the brokenness of their Israelite community. The rape turns into a literary "trope . . . grounded upon a reverence for the female body as a site of the sacred power of life."[185]

Giving full attention to the rape, Keefe deems it a literary element necessary for Israelite authors to imagine a future of wholeness. For Keefe this literary element serves a larger purpose than the literal meaning of rape. Her literary reading, however, devalues the horror of the rape for the woman. Dinah's suffering is but a means to express the political and social struggle of a people. Furthermore, such a metaphorical use suggests that the Israelite narrators reduced the value of women to female bodies. The metaphorical approach is a dangerous approach in a world where "real" rapes happen daily.

Marriage as Solution

In response to Meir Sternberg's positive assessment of the brothers,[186] Danna Nolan Fewell and David M. Gunn present an "alternative reading that is rooted in a somewhat different value system, which we think of as feminist."[187] Contrary to Sternberg's balancing of the rape and the murder, they argue that "the narrator tips the balance in Shechem's favor." They state: "If sympathy is being accumulated, it seems to us to be sympathy for Shechem."[188] Consequently, they dis-

---

[182] Ibid., 84.

[183] Ibid.

[184] Ibid., 94.

[185] Ibid., 88.

[186] See in this chapter the section above "Focus on Men."

[187] Danna Nolan Fewell and David M. Gunn, "Tipping the Balance: Sternberg's Reader and the Rape of Dinah," *Journal of Biblical Literature* 110, no. 2 (1991): 193-211.

[188] Ibid., 197.

like the brothers. "Their [the brothers'] grossly disproportionate response" develops from their sense of injury and stolen honor.[189] If the brothers emerge as heroes, "they are certainly not ours," Fewell and Gunn exclaim.[190]

Distancing themselves from the brothers to sympathize with Shechem, these scholars propose an astonishing alternative: It would have been in Dinah's "best interest within the narrow limits of this society . . . to marry Shechem, the man who loves her and takes delight in her." Fewell and Gunn claim that theirs is a feminist reading because they do not identify Dinah as "a helpless girl to be rescued" but as "a young woman who could have made her own choices—limited though they might have been—had she been asked." Although both scholars acknowledge that "to advocate a woman's marrying her rapist might itself seem to be a dangerous and androcentric advocacy," they argue that "the story world" offers no "other liberating alternatives."[191]

Although Fewell and Gunn are careful to specify the narrow limits of the society from which their alternative emerges, they do not describe the reasons for their reconstruction. Moreover, their view supports a marriage between the rapist and the raped woman according to the terms set by the rapist. Fewell and Gunn allow the hypothesized status quo of the story to direct their interpretation. They do not imagine an alternative because "there would have to be a whole other world." Trapped within patriarchy, their imagination serves patriarchy.

Responding to the critique of Fewell and Gunn, Meir Sternberg, who is not a feminist, reckons that "it is doubtful whether many feminists would underwrite the solution."[192] He estimates that the "marriage-as-solution idea is likely to give offense where it most aims to please: the Women's Liberation movement."[193] Hence, he cautions

---

[189] Ibid., 205, 207.

[190] Ibid., 211.

[191] Ibid., 210.

[192] Meir Sternberg, "Biblical Poetics and Sexual Politics: From Reading to Counterreading," *Journal of Biblical Literature* 111, no. 3 (1992): 475.

[193] Ibid., 478. For a work that questions the suggestion of a marriage between Shechem and Dinah see Burton L. Visotzky, *The Genesis of Ethics: How The Tormented Family of Genesis Leads Us To Moral Development* (New York: Crown, 1996), 199. This interpretation is commendable because the rape is the starting point. However, Visotzky suggests also "that we read the story of Dinah's rape as something that might not be her version of the story" (p. 196). He concedes that "I

Fewell and Gunn: "Tell it not to rapists, publish it not in the streets."[194] In proposing their alternative in the name of feminism, Fewell and Gunn present an interpretation which Sternberg believes, "some would call . . . a license to rape."[195]

In reaction to the interaction among these three scholars Paul Noble suggests a different issue as central in Genesis 34.[196] In contrast to the view of Fewell and Gunn, this story does not try to evoke "appropriate feelings for the story's 'heroes' and 'villains'," but it explores the issue of "crime and punishment" as shown by Sternberg. Noble shows that a basic assumption divides him and Sternberg from Fewell and Gunn. Fewell and Gunn commit to ideological convictions which shape the outcome of their reading. In contrast, Noble posits that like Sternberg he offers his "own interpretation not as yet another 'ideological' reading to be added . . . but to advance . . . towards . . . what *the text itself* says." He insists on the "simply objective, 'hard facts' about the text" that guide him "towards an objective, reader-independent understanding." Therefore, Noble chooses only "from among the alternatives that the text itself offers" by attending carefully to the linguistic details of the narrative. Since "the text omits most of the information we would need to assess Dinah's situation," Noble claims that nothing can be said about her. Consequently, Noble's analysis focuses on the various descriptions of the male characters to show that "*all* the characters are seriously flawed, although they all have some admirable qualities too." Whether Dinah is included in this statement or not remains unclear.

Although Noble describes clearly the epistemological divisions between the two groups of scholars, his proposal does not resolve the dispute. Insisting on the objective standard of linguistic analysis, he rejects the concerns of ideological readers such as Fewell and Gunn. Whereas Noble's essay claims the achievability of objective standards, the history of interpreting Genesis 34 demonstrates its illusiveness.

Irmtraud Fischer likewise considers the marriage proposal an exonerating factor in ancient Israel. Subordinating the narrative to laws in Exodus 22:15-16 and Deuteronomy 22:23-27, she argues that at least

---

do not know how women feminists will react to my . . . reading" but he understands Genesis 34 as "an archetype of the 'girl and boy from opposing tribes fall in love' tale" (p. 196). He proposes two other possible interpretations and concludes by condemning the brothers: "They will forever be doomed to justifying their violence by asking 'Should our sister be made a whore?' " (p. 203).

Shechem tries to restore the legal requirements after the rape. Thus, Shechem does not "brutally" use his power against the other tribe. He has intercourse with Dinah before marrying her, and this is the problem of Genesis 34.

> In der Vergewaltigung [mißachtet Schechem] Recht und Sitte und vor allem die Integrität der Persönlichkeit der Frau. Aber der junge Mann versucht jedoch, diese durch offizielle Heiratsverhandlungen, in denen er sich bereit zeigt, alle Bedingungen anzunehmen, wiederherzustellen.[197]

> By raping, he disregards law and custom and especially the personal integrity of the woman. However, by accepting all conditions, the young man tries to restore them by officially negotiating a marriage.

Shechem is guilty of the rape but he is redeemable. He offers to marry the one whom he raped. Placed within the legal context of marriage negotiations, the problem lies not with the rapist, but rather with the brothers and their "insidious murder."[198] The story exemplifies that marriage negotiations of the family of Sarah and Abraham are often deceptive. When foreign men approach the women of this family, the foreigners and not the "patriarchs" are endangered.

In a later treatment of Genesis 34 Fischer also emphasizes source critical issues. She maintains there that "the later revision places everybody at a disadvantage. Shechem's father becomes greedy, Jacob's sons escalate the revenge. The two young people who are the actual players are both victimized. Not only Dinah but also Shechem become marginalized."[199] Although this approach does not exonerate the rap-

---

[194] Sternberg, "Biblical Poetics," 476.

[195] Ibid., 474.

[196] Paul Noble, "'Balanced' Reading of the Rape of Dinah: Some Exegetical and Methodological Observations," *Biblical Interpretation* 4 (1996): 173-204. The following quotations are from pages 195, 199, 202, and 203.

[197] Irmtraud Fischer, *Die Erzeltern Israels: Feministische-theologische Studien zu Genesis 12-36* (Berlin: de Gruyter, 1994), 233. For other brief references to Genesis 34 see Ann Marmesh, "Anti-Covenant," in *Anti-Covenant: Counter-Reading Women's Lives in the Hebrew Bible*, ed. by Mieke Bal, JSOT Supplement 81: Bible and Literature 22 (Sheffield, UK: Almond Press, 1989), 43-60; Susan Brooks Thistlethwaite, "'You May Enjoy the Spoil of Your Enemies': Rape as a Biblical Metaphor of War," in *Women, War, and Metaphor: Language and Society in the Study of the Hebrew Bible*, ed. Claudia V. Camp and Carole R. Fontaine, Semeia 61 (Atlanta: Scholars Press, 1993), 59-75.

[198] Fischer, *Die Erzeltern Israels*, 232.

[199] Irmtraud Fischer, *Gottesstreiterinnen: Biblische Erzählungen über die Anfänge Israels* (Stuttgart: W. Kohlhammer, 1995), 136.

ist for his deed, the characterization of both Dinah and Shechem as victims still surprises.

The interpretations labeled "feminist" testify to the fluid usage of this adjective. The interpretations do not define it, so that its meaning continues to remain unclear. The analysis showed that a spectrum of views define the label. Some interpreters focus on the redactor, some on the brothers, one on the rape as a metaphor, and several on the marriage as the solution. Indeed, some interpretations, such as the focus on the brothers by Niditch and Rashkow, resemble non-feminist ones, so that the label becomes almost obsolete. This observation also holds for the interpretations of Fewell and Gunn, and Fischer who regard marriage a solution for the rape. The examination of the so-called feminist interpretations demonstrated that—with the exception of Keefe's study—they do not integrate feminist scholarship on rape. They do not focus on the rape or put Dinah into the center. The label "feminist" appears to be based on personal preference, not substantiated by scholarly discourse.

Summary

Genesis 34 chronicles two ethical problems: a rape, and the killing of the rapist and the men of his town. Scholars juggled these two problems, usually emphasizing both or choosing one over the other. The two problems produce questions which many interpretations do not openly acknowledge: Does the rape justify the revengeful killing? What punishment is appropriate for rape? What actually is rape? Is the rapist guilty even when he proposes marriage after the rape? Who is responsible for the events? How should those who are responsible be evaluated? The answers depend on the ideas the interpreters hold about rape.

Interpreters communicate only indirectly their ideas about rape. Scholars consider the brothers as villains and the rapist as a lover. They characterize the relationship between the rape and the revenge by minimizing the rape and stressing the killing. The brothers become outrageous killers; the rapist turns into a loving and acceptable husband for Dinah. The rapist Shechem is credited for his love and the marriage proposal. Even Alice A. Keefe, whose interpretation focuses on the rape, characterizes Shechem as a "passionate young man!"[200]

---

[200] Keefe, *Rapes of Women*, 83.

The analysis of contemporary interpretations has described five foci that marginalized Dinah's rape. First, scholars focused on the male characters to interpret the narrative. Jacob, the brothers, Shechem, or a combination of characters became leading figures. Second, scholars applied source criticism to interpret the story. They reconstructed the original source as a love story which redactors turned into a rape story. Third, scholars characterized Genesis 34 as a story about Israelite tribal history. Individual characters personified Israel's tribes, describing a conflict between the Israelites and the Canaanites. Fourth, interpreters read Genesis 34 as a debate about xenophobia in ancient Israel. The brothers represented the party which favored the exclusion of non-Israelites; Jacob and Dinah represented the party which favored their integration. Fifth, several interpreters labeled their interpretations as feminist. In these interpretations the internal foci varied, but they all marginalized the rape.

Biblical scholars do not present reasons for the marginalization, though several reasons are possible. Some scholars maintained that the narrative itself does not focus on the rape but deals with issues such as tribal history or xenophobia. Immersed in discussions about the tribes of ancient Israel, Gerhard von Rad, for example, identifies the narrative as a personalized version of the "saga" of Shechem. Lyn Bechtel explores possible connections between the anthropological concept of group-oriented societies and ancient Israel in which all activities had to serve the good of the group. In such a society sex outside of boundaries sanctioned by the group was a problem but not rape.

Furthermore, biblical scholars might claim that biblical scholarship deals with the texts themselves and not with issues such as rape. According to this stance interpretations develop from the text (exegesis) and not from outside perspectives (eisegesis). Interpreters stressed that points in their readings of Genesis 34. For instance, Ita Sheres' analysis focuses on the intentionality of the redactors, and she describes their understanding of the story. In other words, she believes to describe what the text or the redactors said. However, the countless examples in this and the previous two chapters demonstrate that there is no text itself, at least not in the case of Genesis 34. The interpreters make the silent text speak, bringing their assumption, their presuppositions, and their cultural understandings of rape to the text. Not the text itself speaks, but the interpreters speak with it. Therefore, text and issues are inseparably intertwined.

In addition, scholars might have marginalized the rape because of textual ambiguity concerning the concept of "love" in the context of rape. Scholars usually assumed that Shechem loved Dinah and trusted his good intentions despite the rape. A critical evaluation of the terminology in the Hebrew text and the resulting meaning in the English could have led them to question the meaning of love. Considering the lasting debates about the meaning of love and its manifestation, they might have been more hesitant to think that love is simply love. In fact, some source critics sensed the potential problem and separated verses accordingly, though without explicit reasoning.

Finally, the marginalization of the rape might be a consequence of the tension between the horror of the rape and the enormity of the killing. Searching for a solution, scholars might have preferred to dismiss the significance of the rape because the killing appeared indefensible. Involving a much greater human cost than the rape of one woman, the rape paled in the mind of interpreters.

Thus, another reading of Genesis 34 will demonstrate that the focus on the rape yields an appropriate interpretation. Informed by feminist scholarship and focused on the rape, Genesis 34 becomes Dinah's story.

Chapter 6

Accentuating Rape:
A Feminist Interpretation
of Dinah's Story

The following exegesis demonstrates that a reader's stance shapes the results of her or his interpretation. Indebted to the discipline of rhetorical criticism,[1] a literary method serves this purpose. The term "rhetorical criticism" was introduced into biblical studies by James Muilenburg in 1968,[2] although the method has a much longer history. As described by Phyllis Trible, rhetorical criticism developed from four areas of literary studies: classical rhetoric, literary critical theory, literary study of the Bible, and form criticism.[3] It emphasizes the final form of the text, proposing that "proper articulation of form-content yields proper articulation of meaning."[4] The repetition of words, phrases, and sentences; the evaluation of different types of discourse; the design and structure of the text; the development of the plot; the portrayal of characters; the features of structure and syntax; and the use of particles—all these are among the literary elements that rhetorical criticism examines. Though this discipline has enlivened biblical scholarship since Muilenburg's formulation, it has not been used for Genesis 34. The application of this method to the text offers, then, new possibilities for the interpretive task.

---

[1] For a description of rhetorical criticism see Phyllis Trible, *Rhetorical Criticism: Context, Method, and the Book of Jonah* (Minneapolis: Fortress, 1994).

[2] James Muilenburg, "Form Criticism and Beyond," *Journal of Biblical Literature* 88 (1969): 1-18.

[3] Trible, *Rhetorical Criticism*, 5.

[4] Ibid., 91.

The method of rhetorical criticism (like any other method) does not itself guarantee a reading that accentuates the rape. As the earlier chapters of this study have demonstrated, the use of a single method does not result in a single interpretation of Genesis 34. Interpreters have applied historical criticism, for example, with varying emphases and results. Some see Genesis 34 as a treatise on xenophobia; some as one of a narrative about tribal history. Some see it as the saga of eponymous ancestors; some as the individual Jacob. Some focus on the brothers and others on Shechem. Furthermore, some historical critics find sources in the narrative and others do not. Some of the former group find two sources, others three. For certain, the single method of historical criticism produces varieties of interpretation. Similarly, the use of rhetorical criticism can be appropriated for diverse interpretations. Here the method is linked to the hermeneutical standpoint of contemporary feminist scholarship on rape.[5]

Literary Overview

In contrast, but not in opposition, to reading Genesis 34 within the Jacob-cycle, this study isolates Genesis 34 from its literary context. Though the values of the former readings are numerous, a restricted reading allows a sustained study of the textual details and the subject of rape. Moreover, the narrative surrounding the text does not yield information about the rape. The two brief references to Dinah in Genesis 30:21 and 46:15 do not relate to chapter 34. They mention Dinah only as the daughter of Leah and Jacob. In the history of interpretation scholars have pursued isolated readings as well as integrated ones.[6] For the purposes of my study the former approach makes the better sense.[7]

---

[5] On the subjectivity of all interpretation see Trible, *Rhetorical Criticism*, 230-33.

[6] For a reading within the Jacob cycle see Michael Fishbane, "Composition and Structure in the Jacob Cycle (Gen. 25:19-35:22)," *Journal of Jewish Studies* 26 (1975): 15-38; Peter L. Lockwood, "Jacob's Other Twin: Reading the Rape of Dinah in Context," *Lutheran Theological Journal* 29 (1995): 98-105. For a reading outside the narrative context see Eduard Nielsen, *Shechem: A Tradition-Historical Investigation* (Copenhagen: Gad, 1955). See also the section "Focus on the Men: Jacob" in chapter 5.

[7] On the issue of isolation of text (as well as integration) the motives may vary. For example, in the history of interpretation scholars have sought to isolate Genesis 34 to minimize its significance in the book of Genesis. By contrast, this study isolates it in order to focus on it and thus to maximize its importance.

A Literary Observation

Although this study isolates Genesis 34 from its surrounding context, the narrative belongs to a body of texts. They constitute the genre of the betrothal type-scene.[8] According to Robert Alter, a betrothal type-scene contains five elements arranged in a fixed pattern.[9] It includes the future bridegroom or his surrogate from a foreign land. There he meets the future bride, the נערה, at a well. She or he draws water, and afterwards she runs home to tell her family about him. The betrothal type-scene ends with a meal between the invited groom and her family. Alter's list of betrothal scenes include: the encounters between Rebekah and Isaac (Genesis 24), Rachel and Jacob (Genesis 29:1-20), the daughters of Reuel and Moses (Exodus 2:15b-21), Ruth and Boaz (book of Ruth), the young women and Saul (1 Samuel 9:11-12), and the Philistine daughter and Samson (Judges 14). As these examples demonstrate variations can occur within the basic pattern. For instance, not every element is always present and the sequence can be changed.

Alter does not include Genesis 34 in his study, but an argument can be made that it belongs to this genre. Like Ruth (Ruth 2:22), Dinah goes out (יצא). Like Rebekah (Genesis 24:14,16), Dinah is called a "young woman" (נערה). Similar to the scene in Samson (Judges 14:5-6), Genesis 34 omits the ritual at the well. Alter argues that instead of this ritual Samson kills a lion—"a pointed substitution for the more decorous and pacific drawing of water from the well."[10] By analogy, instead of meeting Dinah at the well, Shechem rapes Dinah. A ritual of "hostility" substitutes for the "ritual of hospitality."[11] Furthermore, as Samson asks his parents to get him the woman (Judges 14:2), so Shechem asks his father to get him Dinah. According to Alter, the changes depict Samson unfavorably, and so Shechem appears in a poor light. Further similarities emerge between acknowledged betrothal scenes and Genesis 34. During the first meeting Rachel and Jacob do not speak to each other (Genesis 29:9-12). Likewise, Dinah and Shechem do not talk with one another. Ruth does not run home to

---

[8] Genre analysis is a component in the background of rhetorical criticism. For this connection see Trible, *Rhetorical Criticism*, 21-23, 50-51, 81-83, 191-93.

[9] Robert Alter, "Biblical Type-Scenes and the Uses of Convention," chap. in *The Art of Biblical Narrative* (New York: Basic Books, 1981).

[10] Ibid., 61.

[11] Ibid.

Shechem do not talk with one another. Ruth does not run home to bring the news that Boaz, the stranger, arrived (Ruth 2:8-14),[12] and Dinah does not announce Shechem's arrival. Like betrothal scenes, Genesis 34 contains a great deal of kinship language: "the daughter of Leah," "his daughter," "son of Hamor," "sons of Jacob," "their sister," and "their father." All these similarities support the claim that Genesis 34 belongs to the genre of the betrothal scene. In this case, however, the scene has gone awry because the rape has destroyed the potential for a happy outcome.

Building on earlier discussions, Esther Fuchs examines the structure and patriarchal function of betrothal type-scenes and thus adds another important observation. Fuchs maintains that biblical betrothal type-scenes de-emphasize increasingly "the status and the significance of the bride vis-à-vis her future husband, the biblical hero."[13] The genre stresses more and more the groom's "initiation into adult independence and autonomy" whereas the bride's mere transfer "from her father's custody to her husband's custody" reduces her status.[14] Fuchs considers this development a manifestation of "the Bible's patriarchalism."[15] In other words, the genre loses its significance for the divinely appointed heroes of Israel so that, for example, the scenes become gradually shorter. Similar to Alter, Fuchs does not include Genesis 34 into her analysis. If Genesis 34 is included and read as a betrothal type-scene gone awry, a more complex understanding of biblical patriarchalism emerges. Since Genesis 34 presents an aborted version of a betrothal type-scene, it challenges the trend of promoting the groom and devaluing the bride. The story illustrates that rape cannot be tolerated, even by a male hero like Shechem, and so criticizes patriarchal ideology recognizable in other betrothal-type scenes.

---

[12] Although Alter concedes that the whole book of Ruth describes circumstances leading to a betrothal, Ruth 2:8-14 serves as the example. A better proposal would probably refer to chapter 3. Contrary to the element which has the bridegroom arrive in the foreign land, Boaz does not arrive, it is she who arrives in his fields (Ruth 2) and on the threshing floor (Ruth 3).

[13] Esther Fuchs, "Structure and Patriarchal Functions in the Biblical Betrothal Type-Scene: Some Preliminary Notes," *Journal of Feminist Studies in Religion* vol. 3, no. 1 (Spring 1987): 12.

[14] Ibid.

[15] Ibid., 13.

Rhetorical Overview

Genesis 34 is organized into five scenes.[16] The criteria for these are changes in characters and discourse. Scene One: The Rape (vv. 1-3); Scene Two: The Reaction (vv. 4-7); Scene Three: The Negotiations (vv. 8-24); Scene Four: The Killing (vv. 25-29); Scene Five: Jacob and Simeon and Levi (vv. 30-31). Running throughout these scenes are distinctive literary features. The first pertains to the fraternal responses to the rape.[17] Their speech in vv. 14-17 is centrally positioned within the context of all the direct discourses in Genesis 34. Of the seven occurrences, theirs appears in the middle.

1. son Shechem (v. 4)
2. *father Hamor (vv. 8-10)*
3. son Shechem (vv. 11-12)
4. sons of Jacob (vv. 14-17)
5. son Shechem, *father Hamor* (vv. 21-23)
6. *father Jacob (v. 30)*
7. sons of Jacob (v. 31)

This central speech of Dinah's brothers starts and ends with a reference to their sister. Its centrality keeps Dinah present. So the position of their speech refers the reader in a subtle way to the event that necessitated the speech and all the other events of the story.

A second literary feature pertains to the dominance of speeches by all the sons. Shechem, the son of Hamor, has the first word and the brothers, sons of Jacob, the last. Within this large inclusio the pattern repeats itself in smaller units, *mutatis mutandis*. The son Shechem gives the first and third speeches, thus encircling the speech of his father Hamor. Jacob is encircled by the Shechemites on the one side and his sons on the other.

A third literary feature underlines the significance of the rape. Even though Dinah does not speak, the narrative refers continuously to her. In vv. 1-3 every sentence mentions her, once as the subject (v. 1) and

---

[16] Shimon Bar-Efrat, *Narrative Art in the Bible*, Bible and Literature Series 17 (Sheffield, UK: Almond Press, 1989), 96, defines a "scene" the following way: "When all or some of the characters change a new scene starts."

[17] See the detailed analysis of v. 7 in this chapter.

eight times as the object (v. 2a; vv. 2b-3). Thereafter, she continuously appears: Shechem calls her "this young woman" (v. 4); she is "Dinah, his daughter" (v. 5) and the "daughter of Jacob" (vv. 7, 19, cf. v. 3); Hamor mentions her as "your [plural] daughter" and "her" (v. 8); Jacob is "her father" (v. 11); the brothers are "her" brothers (v. 11); she is a "young woman" (v. 12), "Dinah, their sister" (vv. 13, 27); "our sister" (vv. 14, 31) and "our daughter" (v. 17); her brothers are "the brothers of Dinah" (v. 25); and she is simply "Dinah" (v. 26). Though every character in the story refers to Dinah, only the narrator uses her name. She is the main character. The overview of literary features prepares for a close reading of the story.

Close Reading

Scene One: The Rape (vv. 1-3)
Scene One introduces the central characters and reports Shechem's rape of Dinah. The first verse introduces Dinah and her activity.

Verse 1

1 And-went-out Dinah, the-daughter-of Leah	וַתֵּצֵא דִינָה בַּת־לֵאָה
whom she-had-borne to-Jacob	אֲשֶׁר יָלְדָה לְיַעֲקֹב
to-see the-daughters-of the-land.	לִרְאוֹת בִּבְנוֹת הָאָרֶץ׃

The grammatical subject of the sentence is Dinah going out to visit other women in the neighborhood. A single woman planning to visit others represents a rare event in biblical narratives. The introduction of a daughter by her mother's name is rare. Only here and in Genesis 36:39 does a mother's name identify a daughter.[18] Dinah is "the daughter of Leah" and Mehetabel is "the daughter of Matred, daughter of Mezahab." Even in Ruth 1:8 Naomi does not explicitly name the mothers of her two daughters-in-law, Ruth and Orpah: "Go back each of you to your mother's house." In Genesis 34:1 Leah, the mother, is not only named but also the subject of the explicatory relative clause "whom she-had-borne to-Jacob." Rhetorically, Leah links Dinah and

---

[18] For mothers introducing their sons see, e.g., Genesis 24:15: "Bethuel, son of Milcah"; Genesis 24:67: "his mother Sarah"; Genesis 35:23: "the sons of Leah"; Genesis 35:24: "the sons of Rachel . . . the sons of Bilhah"; Genesis 35:25: "the sons of Zilpah."

Jacob. The position of the daughter and the father signifies distance,
an early indication of Jacob's lacking concern for Dinah's well-being.
Women begin and end this verse. One woman, identified by her mother,
hopes to see other women from another people and place. The first
verse promises an unusual story. A very different story from the one
that unfolds is imaginable, one in which women were the main characters. However, the potential for a story in which one woman meets
others disappears quickly. A man sees Dinah and disregards her integrity. The next verse changes Dinah's visit to a nightmare.

Verse 2a

2a But-saw her Shechem,	וַיַּרְא אֹתָהּ שְׁכֶם
the-son-of-Hamor,	בֶּן־חֲמוֹר
the-Hivite,	הַחִוִּי
the-prince-of the-land.	נְשִׂיא הָאָרֶץ

The son of Hamor the Hivite, Shechem appears on the scene. Characterized as the prince of the land, Shechem is of high class. Unlike
Dinah, Shechem is identified by his father rather than by his mother.
He is the son of Hamor. Both father and son are Hivites. Grammatically, the phrase "prince of the land" can refer to Hamor, the nearest
antecedent, or to Shechem, the distant antecedent. In the latter case
Shechem has three identifications: "son of Hamor; the Hivite; the prince
of the land." Later the narrative describes him as someone "most
honored" (v. 19), which made the townspeople listen to him and obey
his request. As the prince of the land, Shechem sees Dinah and uses
his power and position to take what he wants.[19] Plays on the verb "to
see" link the two verses. His action prevents Dinah from seeing the
women of the land. Having been the grammatical subject in v. 1, Dinah
becomes the grammatical object in v. 2. This is the position into which
Shechem forces her. To see her leads to her rape. Ironically, his seeing of Dinah will prevent her from seeing the women of the land. His
intention is hostile. The violence begins.

---

[19] Bruce Vawter acknowledges this interpretation in *On Genesis: A New Reading* (Garden City, NY: Doubleday, 1977), 357: "The local squire, used to taking
what he wants when and where he finds it, oppresses a comely peasant girl." How
Vawter knows she is a peasant girl remains unclear. After all, her father is of high
stature himself.

Verses 2b-3

2b And-he-took her,	וַיִּקַּח אֹתָהּ
and-he-laid-her,	וַיִּשְׁכַּב אֹתָהּ
and-he-raped-her.	וַיְעַנֶּהָ:
3 and-remained-close he to-Dinah, the-daughter-of Jacob	וַתִּדְבַּק נַפְשׁוֹ בְּדִינָה בַּת־יַעֲקֹב
and-he-lusted-after the-young-women,	וַיֶּאֱהַב אֶת־הַנַּעֲרָ
and-he-spoke to-the-heart-of the-young-woman.	וַיְדַבֵּר עַל־לֵב הַנַּעֲרָ:

No references to time and place delay the actions.[20] Grammatically, Shechem is the subject and Dinah the object. Six verbs in rapid succession describe them.[21] The first three report rape, the last three its ramification.

The first set of verbs. In staccato fashion, the narrative combines the first three verbs with pronouns to describe the rape: "he-took-her, and-he-laid-her, and-he-raped-her" (v. 2b). These verbs underscore the increasing severity of the violence.[22] Whereas the first verb, לקח, means simply "to take," the second, שכב, presents an interesting twist. The verb is not connected to the expected preposition את (with) but to the object marker אות. It stresses the grammatical position of Dinah as the object of the activity.[23] Shechem does not lie "with" her. The marker indicates that Shechem acted without regard for Dinah. He is the subject of the verb, and she the object. Dinah does not consent. No doubt, "Shechem laid her."

The Septuagint does not reflect this obvious meaning, despite the evidence of the Masoretic Text. Preferring the preposition, the Greek translation suggested that Dinah consented: "Shechem laid with (μετ'

---

[20] See Shimon Bar-Efrat, "Time and Space," chap. in *Narrative Art in the Bible*, Bible and Literature Series 17 (Sheffield, UK: Sheffield Academic Press, 1989), 141ff.

[21] The use of six verbs in such a relationship is characteristic of biblical speech, e.g., Genesis 22:3-4; 2 Samuel 13:8c-9b; Jonah 1:15-16 passim.

[22] For this evaluation see Nahum M. Sarna, *Genesis: The Traditional Hebrew Text with New JPS Translation*, JPS Torah Commentary Series (Philadelphia: Jewish Publication Society, 1989), 234.

[23] Recent grammarians regard the particle also as a marker of emphasis when a noun joins it. Such an understanding supports the interpretation that the narrative stresses Dinah as the object of the activity. When the particle appears with the nominative, grammarians are uncertain about its function, cf. Bruce K. Waltke and M. O'Connor, *An Introduction to Biblical Hebrew Syntax* (Winona Lake, Indiana: Eisenbrauns, 1990), 177-78.

'αυτής) Dinah." At stake is the gravitiy of rape.[24] Other biblical rape stories do not support the translation of שכב with a preposition. Interpreting the story about the rape of Tamar by Amnon (2 Samuel 13), J. P. Fokkelman maintained that in v. 14 the verb and object marker (את שכב) described "clearly the sexual act of violence of which Amnon is the subject and Tamar the objectivized, depersonalized victim."[25] Similarly, in Genesis 34:2, Dinah is "the objectivized, depersonalized victim" and Shechem is "the subject."

The third verb, ענה in the piel, also poses a problem. Some scholars argued that it does not translate as "to rape."[26] Classical reference books indicated, however, that ענה signifies an act of violence. For example, the concordance of Mandelkern offered the Latin equivalent "*opprimere, vim affere*,"[27] which refers to violent and oppressive action.[28] Francis Brown, S. R. Driver, and Charles A. Briggs translated the verb as "1. humble, mishandle, afflict; 2. humble, a woman by cohabitation; 3. afflict; 4. humble, weaken."[29] Wilhelm Gesenius translated the verb as "to weaken a woman, through rape."[30] These refer-

---

[24] August Dillmann suggested that the preposition is the "rougher" expression, see his *Die Genesis,* für die 3. Auflage nach Dr. August Knobel, kurzgefasstes exegetisches Handbuch zum Alten Testament, eilfte Lieferung, 6th ed. (Leipzig: S. Hirzel, 1892), 372: "Wenn ihre [der Masoreten] Überlieferung richtig ist, so ist offenbar שכב את (eine beschlafen) der gröbere Ausdruck, u. hier (wie 2 S. 13, 14), wo es um Nothzucht handelt, ganz am Platz." See also Franz J. Delitzsch, *Neuer Commentar über die Genesis,* 5th ed. (Leipzig: Dörffling und Franke, 1887), 414; Victor P. Hamilton, *The Book of Genesis: Chapters 18-50,* The New International Commentary on the Old Testament (Grand Rapids, MI: Eerdmans, 1995), 354.

[25] J. P. Fokkelman, *Narrative Art and Poetry in the Books of Samuel,* vol. 1 (Assen, Netherlands: Van Gorcum, 1981), 105.

[26] See, for example, Lyn M. Bechtel, "What If Dinah Is Not Raped? (Genesis 34)," *Journal for the Study of Old Testament* 62 (1994): 19-36; see also chapters 3 and 5 of this book.

[27] Solomon Mandelkern, *Veteris Testamenti Concordantiae Hebraicae atque Chaldaicae* (Tel Aviv: Schocken, 1967), 902.

[28] See P. G. W. Glare, ed., *Oxford Latin Dictionary,* vol. 2 (Oxford, UK: Clarendon Press, 1973), 1257: "opprimo" no. 1-7; P. G. W. Glare, ed., *Oxford Latin Dictionary,* vol. 1 (Oxford, UK: Clarendon Press, 1968), 78: "affero," no. 9.

[29] Francis Brown, S. R. Driver, and Charles A. Briggs, eds., *Hebrew and English Lexicon of the Old Testament, based on the Lexicon of William Gesenius* (Oxford: Oxford University Press, 1951), 776.

[30] Wilhelm Gesenius, *Hebräisches und Aramäisches Handwörterbuch über das Alte Testament* (Berlin: Springer, 1962), 604: "ein Weib schwächen, durch Notzucht."

ence books understood that the verb described a form of violent interaction, including rape.[31]

Several contemporary scholars support this understanding. For
example, the biblical scholar Moshe Weinfeld suggests—rather unin-
tentionally—to translate the verb as "to rape" when he discusses
Deuteronomy 22:13-29. Although he states that the verb ענה
"connote[s] sexual intercourse in general rather than rape,"[32] he later
holds that "the author of Deuteronomy does not differentiate between
cases of seduction and rape" because "sexual relations with a young,
even unbetrothed, girl had always been taken as coercive."[33] In other
words, men in the ancient Near East forced young women to have
intercourse, which equals the meaning of the verb "to rape." Despite
Weinfeld's attempt to suggest otherwise, his explanations indicate the
meaning "to rape" for the verb ענה. Erhard S. Gerstenberger also translates the piel of ענה as "to rape." He states that ענה describes "unjust
situations," "the creation of a miserable situation"[34] and "physical or
psychological violence."[35]

In conclusion of v. 2b, the three verbs יקח, שׁכב (את), and ענה function on two levels of meaning. The verbs can be treated similarly to
the rhetorical device of hendiadys, a feature of Hebrew syntax in which
two words are used to describe one activity.[36] Here the three verbs
connected by conjunctions express the single action of rape. The use
of this device underscores the act. On another level the three words
suggest a progressive severity. They emphasize Shechem's increasing
use of violence against Dinah in v. 2b.

The second set of verbs. Three verbs report the immediate consequences of the rape. The first is דבק, combined with the pronoun ב

---

[31] Other biblical texts use the verb ענה in the piel, e.g., Lamentations 5:11: "Women
are raped in Zion" (NRSV). For contemporary scholars who support this translation
see passim in chapter 5. Cf. Robert Alter, *Genesis* (New York: W. W. Norton, 1996)
who translates Genesis 34:2 as "he debased her." This archaic expression seems to
evaluate rape from the perspective of those who believed that women lose their
value through rape.

[32] Moshe Weinfeld, *Deuteronomy and the Deuteronomistic School* (Oxford:
Clarendon Press, 1972), 286.

[33] Ibid., 287 n. 3.

[34] Erhard S. Gerstenberger, "ענה 'anah," in *Theologisches Wörterbuch zum Alten
Testament*, ed. Heinz-Josef Fabry and Helmer Ringgren, vol. 6 (Stuttgart:
Kohlhammer, 1989), 252.

[35] Ibid., 253.

[36] Thomas O. Lamdin, *Introduction to Biblical Hebrew* (New York: Charles
Scribner's Sons, 1971), 238-40.

and the noun נפש. The verb is often translated as "to love."[37] Based
on the use of דבק in other biblical passages, an alternative translation
is possible. For example, in Ruth 1:14 the verb connotes spatial closeness. The verse describes that Ruth and Naomi stayed together while
the other daughter-in-law left for home: "But Ruth clung to [דבק ב]
her" (RSV). The Jerusalem Bible translated the verse more clearly as a
reference to spatial closeness, "Ruth stayed with [דבק ב] Naomi." The
verb also appears in Ruth 2:23, which the RSV translated as such a
reference: "So she kept close to [דבק ב] the maidens of Boaz" and the
NRSV: "So she stayed close to [דבק ב] the young women of Boaz."

Describing the spatial distance between the lover and the hater of
God, Psalm 101:3 uses the phrase דבק ב with the meaning "to stay
close." According to commentator A. A. Anderson, the verb דבק with
the pronoun ב denotes "to keep close to someone."[38] Thus, he translated Psalm 101:3: "It shall not cleave to me: or 'he shall not remain
close to me.'"[39] Two verses in Numbers 36 contain the verb [ב] דבק.
The NRSV translated Numbers 36:7, "For all Israelites shall retain
[דבק ב] the inheritance of their ancestral tribes," and Numbers 36:9,
"For each of the tribes of the Israelites shall retain [דבק ב] its own
inheritance." Already Gesenius proposed the translation: "to keep something (possession)."[40] The verb indicates physical and spatial but not
emotional closeness.

In v. 3 the grammatical subject of the verb דבק is the noun נפש.
Often mistranslated as "soul," the noun נפש originally signified the
throat and paraphrases personal pronouns in numerous texts,[41] for

---

[37] See, e.g., Bechtel, "What if Dinah," 29; George W. Coats, *Genesis with an
Introduction to Narrative Literature*, FOTL; Grand Rapids, MI: Eerdmans, 1983),
234; Gerhard von Rad, *Genesis: A Commentary* (Philadelphia: Westminster Press,
1972), 331.

[38] A. A. Anderson, *The Book of Psalms*, New Century Bible, vol. 2 (London:
Marshall, Morgan & Scott, 1972), 458.

[39] Ibid., vol. 1, 702.

[40] Gesenius, *Handwörterbuch*, 152: "an einem Besitz festhalten."

[41] See H. Seebaß, "נפש naepaes," in *Theologisches Wörterbuch zum Alten
Testament*, ed. Heinz-Josef Fabry and Helmer Ringgren, vol. 5 (Stuttgart:
Kohlhammer, 1986), 531. For an appendix on the translation of "soul" see ibid.,
543-45. See also Hans Walter Wolff, *Anthropologie des Alten Testaments* (München:
Kaiser, 1977), 25-48; Claus Westermann, "נפש naefaes," in *Theologisches
Handwörterbuch zum Alten Testament*, ed. Ernst Jenni and Claus Westermann,
vol. 2 (München: Kaiser, 1976), 71-96, esp. 75: "An einer Reihe von Stellen hat
naefaes die Bedeutung 'Gier, Begier, Verlangen.' Diese Gruppe steht der Bed. 'Kehle,

example in Genesis 49:6, Numbers 32:10, Jeremiah 16:30 and Psalm
25:13.[42] The phrase ותדבק נפשו בדינה in Genesis 34:3 thus simply
reads: "He stayed close to Dinah."⌐

Another translation of נפש is possible. Brown, Driver, and Briggs
translated נפש as the "seat of emotions and passions: desire."[43] Accordingly, the phrase would translate as "his desire remained close to
Dinah," referring to Shechem's "volitional appetite."[44] This understanding of נפש describes clearly the sexually objectifying dimension of
Shechem's motives, and is therefore preferred. The phrase then reads:
"His desire remained close to Dinah, the daughter of Jacob."⌐

Within the context of rape the second verb of v. 3, אהב, does not
simply mean to "love." Rather, it describes Shechem's intention after
the rape to treat Dinah as he pleases. Two scholarly observations support such an understanding of אהב. G. Wallis stated: "The terminological context for to love/love is very wide in the language of the Old
Testament."[45] Since "love and action are two sides of the same coin,"[46]
concrete action fills the meaning of "love." Interpreting the rape of
Tamar in 2 Samuel 13, Phyllis Trible discusses this verb. Care and
support do not define its meaning but rather the "ambiguous word 'to
desire', to let the plot disclose the precise meaning."[47] A similar definition guides the translation of Genesis 34:3. In the context of rape the
verb does not refer to mutual intimacy. Rather, it indicates the mean-

---

Schlund' am nächsten; weder die Übersetzung 'Seele' noch 'Leben' wäre hier möglich.
n. ist hier die Kraft des Verlangens, die aus dem Leersein der Kehle, des Rachens
entsteht, wobei aber die Kraft des Verlangens über Hunger und Durst hinaus erweitert
ist." For a classic discussion see Johs. Pedersen, "The Soul, Its Powers and Capacity," chap. in *Israel: Its Life and Culture*, vol. I-II (London: Cumberlege, 1926;
reprint 1959), 99-181.

[42] Seebaß, "נפש naepaes," 660.

[43] Brown, Driver, and Briggs, *Hebrew and English Lexicon of the Old Testament*, 660.

[44] #1395 נפש (nepesh)," in *Theological Wordbook of the Old Testament*, ed.
R. Laird Harris, Gleason L. Archer, and Bruce K. Waltke, vol. 2 (Chicago: Moody,
1980), 588; see also Seebaß, "נפש naepaes," 540.

[45] G. Wallis, "אהב 'ahab," in *Theologisches Wörterbuch zum Alten Testament*,
ed. Heinz-Josef Fabry and Helmer Ringgren, vol. 1 (Stuttgart: Kohlhammer, 1973),
111: "Das Begriffsfeld lieben/Liebe ist im alttestamentlichen Idiom sehr weit
gespannt."

[46] Ibid., 115: "Liebe und Handeln sind die beiden Seiten der gleichen Münze."

[47] Phyllis Trible, "Tamar: The Royal Rape of Wisdom," chap. in *Texts of Terror:
Literary-Feminist Readings of Biblical Narratives* (Philadelphia: Fortress, 1984),
58, footnote 6.

ing "to desire" in the sense of "to lust (after)." As Amnon lusted after
Tamar before he raped her, so Shechem raped Dinah before he lusted
after her. In Genesis 34 the verb has lost its "ambiguity" because the
rape preceded his perverse lust. The verb אהב expresses Shechem's
interest to exert his will for sex over Dinah.

The third verb, דבר, appears in the phrase דבר על לב and describes
Shechem's attempt to make Dinah compliant. He has to calm her
because she did not consent. Whereas many translations read the phrase
דבר על לב as "he spoke tenderly to her" (NRSV), Georg Fischer proposed that דבר על לב means "to try to talk against a negative opinion"
or "to change a person's mind."[48] The phrase occurs ten times throughout the Hebrew Bible: Genesis 34:3 and 50:21, Judges 19:3, 1 Samuel
1:13, 2 Samuel 19:8, Isaiah 40:2, Hosea 2:16, Ruth 2:13, and 2
Chronicles 30:22 and 32:6. The phrase appears when "the situation
is wrong, difficult, or danger is in the air."[49] Someone speaks to the
"heart" of the fearful character to resolve a frightening situation in a
larger context of fear, anxiety, sin, or offense; when someone tries to
"talk against a prevailing (negative) opinion."[50] In the context of Genesis 34, the phrase describes Shechem's attempts to change Dinah's
negative opinion and to make her accept his interests. The phrase
thus reads: "He attempted to soothe the young woman."

[This interpretation of Genesis 34:1-3 indicates that several verbs
describe the selfishness and the disregard Shechem held for Dinah.
Expressing the sheer power and dominance of the rape, the first scene
turns the woman from subject to object. She does not even speak.
The scene shows also that the rapist attempts immediately to hide his
deed. Shechem tries to "soothe" Dinah. Feminist scholarship discloses
that rapists often try to appear "normal" after the rape, especially in
situations of acquaintance rape. Differentiating between "hostility rape"
and "sexual gratification rape," feminist scholars explain that the latter is the more ambiguous and confused one.[51] The rapist is not likely
to brutalize the woman. He will threaten and overpower her but not
resort to murder or beating. The man sees women as objects. Such a

---

[48] The basis of the following analysis is Georg Fischer, "Die Redewendung
דבר על לב im AT—Ein Beitrag zum Verständnis von Jes 40,2," *Biblica* 65 (1984):
244-50.

[49] Ibid., 249.

[50] Ibid., 250.

[51] Andra Medea and Kathleen Thompson, *Against Rape* (New York: Farrar, Straus
& Giroux, 1974), 21.

rapist knows that he takes advantage of the woman because he does not pay or compensate her. He might even contact her again after the rape and pretend that nothing wrong happened.[52] Understood as a "sexual gratification rapist," Shechem considered Dinah an "opportunity" when she walked to meet the daughters of the land. The interpretation confirms the notion of feminist scholarship that rape is sexual violence. When rape is accentuated, love talk is not involved.

Scene Two: The Reaction (vv. 4-7)

The rape has occurred. Society reacts, and the aftermath begins. Scene Two offers neither an explicit response from Dinah nor a report of Shechem going home to his father. But the four verses describe the different reactions of the two families. Like flashlight beams, the verses jump from family to family. In an alternating fashion, vv. 4 and 6 refer to the reaction of Shechem and his father Hamor whereas vv. 5 and 7 describe the reaction of Jacob and his sons. Crisscrossing incidents[53] begin with Shechem's family but end with Dinah's family.

Verses 4-7

4 Then-said <u>Shechem</u> to Hamor, his-father: וַיֹּאמֶר שְׁכֶם אֶל־חֲמוֹר אָבִיו לֵאמֹר
   Take for-me the-young-woman the-this as-a wife.   *קַח־לִי אֶת־הַיַּלְדָּה הַזֹּאת לְאִשָּׁה׃*

5 And-Jacob heard   וְיַעֲקֹב שָׁמַע
      that he-had-oppressed <u>Dinah, his-daughter</u>;   כִּי טִמֵּא אֶת־דִּינָה בִתּוֹ
      and-his-sons were-with-his-cattle on-the-field,   וּבָנָיו הָיוּ אֶת־מִקְנֵהוּ בַּשָּׂדֶה
      and-kept-silent Jacob until *they-came.*   וְהֶחֱרִשׁ יַעֲקֹב עַד־בֹּאָם׃
6 Went-out Hamor, the-father-of <u>Shechem</u>, to Jacob   וַיֵּצֵא חֲמוֹר אֲבִי־שְׁכֶם אֶל־יַעֲקֹב
      to-speak to-him.   לְדַבֵּר אִתּוֹ׃
7 And-the-sons-of Jacob *came* from-the-field,   וּבְנֵי יַעֲקֹב בָּאוּ מִן־הַשָּׂדֶה
      when-<u>they-heard</u>,   כְּשָׁמְעָם
   and-grieved the-men   וַיִּתְעַצְּבוּ הָאֲנָשִׁים
   and-it-and- it-was-depressed to-them much   וַיִּחַר לָהֶם מְאֹד
      because disorder he-did in-Israel   כִּי־נְבָלָה עָשָׂה בְיִשְׂרָאֵל
      to-lay <u>the-daughter-of</u> Jacob   לִשְׁכַּב אֶת־בַּת־יַעֲקֹב
   and-so not <u>it-was-done.</u>[54]   וְכֵן לֹא יֵעָשֶׂה׃

---

[52] Ibid., 26.

[53] Bar-Efrat, *Narrative Art*, 95, defines an "incident" as "the smallest narrative unit."

[54] The series of markers signals associations among words, phrases, clauses, and sentences and supports the exegesis. For this system see Trible, *Rhetorical Criticism*, 105.

Interestingly, the name of the rapist Shechem appears in his family sections but not in Dinah's family. The narrator introduces Shechem's speech to his father Hamor. It is the first direct speech in the story.

Verse 4

4 Then-said Shechem to Hamor, his-father: וַיֹּאמֶר שְׁכֶם אֶל־חֲמוֹר אָבִיו לֵאמֹר
   Take for-me the-young-woman the-this as-a wife. קַח־לִי אֶת־הַיַּלְדָּה הַזֹּאת לְאִשָּׁה׃

The places have changed, time has passed, and a new character appears. Hamor, the father of Shechem, is on stage with Shechem and perhaps Dinah. The demonstrative pronoun זאת hints at her presence. The raped young woman stands before the father of the rapist. Without mentioning the rape, Shechem requests that Hamor proceed with a marriage arrangement. He uses the same verb for this request that the narrator used to describe the rape: "take." Shechem does not name Dinah. He refers to her only as ילדה,"young woman." This noun appears only two other times in biblical literature[55] and signifies a sexually mature young woman.[56] Shechem gives no reason for his request. He speaks but six terse words. The incident switches to Dinah's family. Jacob, the father, hears about the rape.

Verse 5

5 And-Jacob heard   וַיַּעֲקֹב שָׁמַע
         that he-had-oppressed Dinah, his-daughter;   כִּי טִמֵּא אֶת־דִּינָה בִתּוֹ
   and-his-sons were with-his-cattle on-the-field,   וּבָנָיו הָיוּ אֶת־מִקְנֵהוּ בַּשָּׂדֶה
   and-kept-silent Jacob until they-came.   וְהֶחֱרִשׁ יַעֲקֹב עַד־בֹּאָם׃

The narrated report does not disclose the details as to how Jacob received the news. How did anybody know? Introduced by the particle כי, the phrase "he-had-oppressed (טמא) Dinah, his-daughter" is the key to the sentence. The verb טמא is also a key verb in the story (cf. vv. 13, 27). A typical term of the priestly tradition, טמא often appears

---

[55] Joel 4:3, Zacharia 8:5. See Solomon Mandelkern, *Veteris Testamenti Concordantiae Hebraicae atque Chaldaicae* (Tel Aviv: Schocken, 1967).

[56] See "#867 ילד (yalad)," in *Theological Wordbook,* vol. 1, 867: These words are generally used for very young children but sometimes refer to adolescents and even young adults." See also Benno Jacob, *Das Erste Buch der Tora* (Berlin: Schocken, 1934), 650, 653, who interprets ילדה as "Mädel," a term he considers "burschikos" (hoydenish) and "intim" (intimate) without offering further proof.

in Leviticus, Numbers, and Ezekiel.[57] It relates to cultic impurity. Many interpretations of this verse appeal to that tradition. For example, Brueggemann writes that "the woman is not simply taken. She is made ritually unacceptable."[58] In this understanding the uncleanliness affects Dinah's status.[59] She, not the rapist, becomes "ritually unacceptable."

Besides the meaning of טמא found in the priestly tradition, the verb has a political-ethical meaning in two prophetic texts. In Micah 2:10 the root טמא refers to the injustice and oppression of powerful rulers in Judah: "Arise and go; for this is no place to rest, because of uncleanliness (טָמְאָה) that destroys with a grievous destruction" (NRSV). In the prediction, God announces through the prophet Micah that the rulers of Judah will be punished for their "uncleanness." The term, however, does not refer to ritual uncleanliness but to the taking of the fields (Micah 2:2), the oppression of householder and house (Micah 2:2), the stealing from the peaceful (Micah 2:8), and the evacuation of poor people from their houses (Micah 2:9).[60]

---

[57] For example see Leviticus 13:3, 22, 27, 44; 20:3, 25; Numbers 5:2, 6:7; 19:19, Ezekiel 5:11; 9:7; 18:6, 11, 15; 22:11; 33:26. On the meaning of this verb see Tikva Frymer-Kensky, "The Strange Case of the Suspected Sotah (Num. 5.11-31)," *Vetus Testamentum* 34, no. 1 (1984): 11-26. For further discussions on טמא see Jacob Milgrom, *Leviticus 1-16: A New Translation*, The Anchor Bible (New York; Doubleday, 1991).

[58] Walter Brueggemann, *Genesis: A Bible Commentary for Teaching and Preaching* (Atlanta: Knox Press, 1982), 376.

[59] For the assumed connection between uncleanliness and sin see, for example, Helmer Ringgren, *Israelitische Religion*, 2d rev. ed. (Stuttgart: Kohlhammer, 1982), 128.

[60] Doubting that Micah 2:10 uses טמא in a political-ethical sense, interpreters changed the root of the verb, see G. André, "טמא tame,'" in *Theologisches Wörterbuch zum Alten Testament*, ed. Heinz-Josef Fabry and Helmer Ringgren, vol. 3 (Stuttgart: Kohlhammer, 1982), 364, who writes that the use of the verb is "eigenartig" [peculiar] in Micah 2:10, "da sonst nirgendwo Unterdrückung als Unreinheit bezeichnet wird" [because nowhere else is oppression called uncleanliness]. Scholars proposed to change the word to מְאוּמָה (anything); see, for example, Arnold B. Ehrlich, *Randglossen zur Hebräischen Bibel: Textkritisches, Sprachliches und Sachliches*, vol. 5 (Leipzig: Hinrich, 1912), 1912. For another proposal see Hans Walter Wolff, *Micha: A Commentary*, trans. Gary Stansell (Minneapolis: Augsburg, 1990), 71: "MT ('unclean') should be taken as a *qal* infinitive (*tom'a*) used as a noun; however, since this would be entirely without parallel, perhaps the word should be vocalized as the usual noun טָמְאָה."

The second text is Hosea 6:10: "In the house of Israel I have seen
a horrible thing; Ephraim's whoredom is there, Israel is defiled (נִטְמָא)"
(NRSV). Wilhelm Rudolph comments:

> Und wenn das alles zuletzt Hurerei und *Unreinheit* genannt wird (V. 10b), so
> macht das nur wieder einmal wahr, daß sich die Untreue gegen Jahwe nicht
> bloß auf dem religiösen, sondern ganz unmittelbar auf dem *sittlichen* Gebiet
> auswirkt.[61] [stress added]

> And if all this is called whoredom and *uncleanliness* (v. 10b), it shows again
> that unfaithfulness against Yahwe affects not only the religious but also the
> *ethical* realm.

In this text the root טמא refers to a setting beyond ritual and cultic
uncleanliness. "Unfaithfulness" toward God reaches into the realm of
ethics. When injustice and oppression rule, they make Israel morally
"unclean." The social and political order requires "cleansing."

Understood in this prophetic context, the root טמא in Genesis 34:5
expresses the oppressive and unjust nature of the rape. It brings oppression and injustice to Dinah and her family, and so it extends beyond "ritual" uncleanliness. The situation cries out for the reestablish-
ment of the social and political order that requires redress.

In v. 5, the male characters appear in parallel structures ABA'B':

<u>Jacob</u> (A) hears . . . but the *sons* (B) are in the field.
<u>Jacob</u> (A') keeps silent until *they* (B') come.

Jacob is the first to hear the news; the sons appear last in the parallelism. This location emphasizes them to suggest their increasing importance. Whereas Jacob responded with silence, their reaction is still to
come.

Like Jacob, father of Dinah, Hamor, father of Shechem does not
keep the expected dominant role. Both fathers become mediators for
their active sons. The sons start and end Scene Two. Arranged
chiastically, the references in v. 4 and v. 5 to sons and fathers demonstrate this pattern. In v. 4 son Shechem (A) speaks to father Hamor
(B). In v. 5 father Jacob (B') hears, reacts with silence, and waits for
the return of his sons (A'). Though the response of Jacob's sons would
seem to be the next logical step, v. 6 returns to Hamor.

---

[61] Wilhelm Rudolph, *Hosea*, Kommentar zum Alten Testament Series, vol. 13
(Gütersloh: Gütersloher Verlagshaus, 1966), 145.

Verse 6

6 Went-out Hamor, the-father-of Shechem, to Jacob	וַיֵּצֵא חֲמוֹר אֲבִי־שְׁכֶם אֶל־יַעֲקֹב
to-speak to-him.	לְדַבֵּר אִתּוֹ:

This topic returns to the incident in v. 4. Hamor complies with the request of his son. One father addresses the other. As Dinah went out in v. 1, Hamor goes out here. Her goal was to visit the daughters of the land; his is to secure her for marriage. The story does not say that Hamor knows about the rape. Motivations and intentions remain unspoken. As the ruler of the land, Hamor might be inclined to hide the crime of his son if he knew about it. But if not, he would negotiate in good faith.

While Hamor is on his way, the narrative returns to Jacob's family. This interruption of the preceding incident creates tension. The different characters pass quickly in front of the reader's eyes. The narrative returns to the brothers of Dinah. Their delayed but expected response is described in detail:

Verse 7

7 And-the-sons-of Jacob came from the-field,	וּבְנֵי יַעֲקֹב בָּאוּ מִן־הַשָּׂדֶה
when-they-heard,	כְּשָׁמְעָם
and-grieved the-men	וַיִּתְעַצְּבוּ הָאֲנָשִׁים
and-it-and- it-was-depressed to-them much	וַיִּחַר לָהֶם מְאֹד
because disorder he-did in-Israel	כִּי נְבָלָה עָשָׂה בְיִשְׂרָאֵל
to-lay the-daughter-of Jacob	לִשְׁכַּב אֶת־בַּת־יַעֲקֹב
and-so not it-was-done.[54]	וְכֵן לֹא יֵעָשֶׂה:

Paired with v. 5 this verse repeats its vocabulary of שמע, שדה, בוא. In both verses the particle כי signals the importance of what follows.[62] In v. 5 Jacob keeps silent until the sons "come;" in v. 7 the sons "come" when they hear. In v. 5 the sons are with the cattle in the "field;" in v. 7 the sons came from the "field." In v. 5 Jacob "heard" that Dinah had been "oppressed;" in v. 7 the sons "hear." The relationship of these three words in the two verses forms a chiasm. In

---

[62] See the Hebrew text of v. 5 quoted earlier in this chapter.

v. 5 Jacob <u>hears</u> (A), the sons are in the *field* (B), and they will <u>*come*</u> (C); in v. 7 the sons <u>*come*</u> (C') from the *field* (B') when they <u>hear</u> (A'). In v. 5 the particle כִּי introduces the relative clause about Dinah's "oppression;" in v. 7 it introduces the reason for the fraternal response. In addition to having verbal repetitions, vv. 5 and 7 share two related concepts, oppression (טמא) and disorder (נְבָלָה).

Verse 7 is a long verse. Based on grammatical features, it can be divided into three sections. The first section reiterates that the brothers come from the field. Here the subject of the sentence is emphasized because the Hebrew places the subject (בְּנֵי יַעֲקֹב the sons of Jacob) in front of the verb (בָּאוּ they came).

And-the-sons-of Jacob came from the-field,	וּבְנֵי יַעֲקֹב בָּאוּ מִן־הַשָּׂדֶה
when-they-heard	כְּשָׁמְעָם

The second section describes the emotional response of the brothers. It comes in two clauses with two imperfect consecutive verbs.

and-grieved the-men	וַיִּתְעַצְּבוּ הָאֲנָשִׁים
and-it-was-depressed to-them much.	וַיִּחַר לָהֶם מְאֹד

The first verb, עצב, appears in the Hitpa'el. Only one other biblical text, Genesis 6:6, uses the verb with this stem. There God reacts to the evil of humankind with grief: "and it grieved him [Yhwh] to his heart" (NRSV). Interpreters underline the depth and profundity of divine grief in this passage. U. Cassuto writes, "Man's deeds and the thoughts of his heart (v. 5) bring grief to the *heart* of the Lord."[63] Nahum Sarna states that "God's decision is made in sorrow not in anger."[64] Brueggemann offers one of the most elaborate explanations in Genesis 6:6: "Verse 6 shows us the deep pathos of God. God is not angered but grieved. He is not enraged but saddened." Further, the "narrative is centered in the grief of God. What distinguishes God in this narrative from every other god and from every creature is God's deep grief. That grief enables God to move past his own interest."[65] Relating this understanding of עצב to Genesis 34:7 deepens the inter-

[63] U. Cassuto, *A Commentary on the Book of Genesis*, trans. I. Abrahams, Part I: *From Adam to Noah Gen 1-6.8* (Jerusalem: Magnes Press, Hebrew University Press, 1978), 304.

[64] Sarna, *Genesis*, 47.

[65] Brueggemann, *Genesis*, 77, 78, 82.

pretation of the fraternal response. As God grieved over the creation, so the brothers grieve for Dinah's rape.

The second verb, חרה, adds another dimension to the fraternal response. Here the grief of the brothers influences the meaning. In Genesis 6:6 God's grief influences God's repentance.[66] The verb is joined by the preposition ל. Although scholars often render the verb as "to be angry, to burn," Mayer I. Gruber presents strong evidence for a different translation. He observes that the expression (חרה (ל is often confused with (חרה (אף and translated as "to be angry." An examination "of the other twenty-two attestations of Heb. (חרה (ל reveals that in at least eleven cases this expression denotes 'became depressed.'"[67] The translation "to be depressed" depicts the internally directed sadness about the rape, while the translation "to be angry" refers to the externally directed aggressive sadness. Since the externally directed response of the brothers appears later in the narrative, the translation "to be depressed" is appropriate here. It indicates the deep interior response of the brothers.

An interesting parallel to this response appears in Genesis 45:5. Both verbs, עצב (Niphal) and (חרה (ל describe the grief of Joseph's brothers. Scholars propose that the parallelism of the verb חרה with עצב underlines the theological significance of the response. This verse is part of "the center and focus of the Joseph narrative."[68] Although Genesis 34:7 is not explicitly theological, the parallel suggests the depth of the grief and depression the brothers felt about the rape of their sister. No characters in the story reveal such a profound reaction to the rape.

The third section, beginning with the particle כִּי, offers the reason for the depth of the fraternal response.

because disorder he-did in-Israel	כִּי נְבָלָה עָשָׂה בְיִשְׂרָאֵל
to-lay the-daughter-of Jacob	לִשְׁכַּב אֶת־בַּת־יַעֲקֹב
and-so not it-was-done.	וְכֵן לֹא יֵעָשֶׂה:

---

[66] The influence of עצב on God's repentance in Genesis 6:6 is pointed out by C. F. Keil and F. Delitzsch, *Biblical Commentary on the Old Testament*, vol. 1: *The Pentateuch*, trans. James Martin (Grand Rapids, MI: Eerdmans, 1949), 139f: "The form of יִנָּחֶם it *repented* the Lord,' may be gathered from the explanatory יִתְעַצֵּב, 'it grieved him at His heart.' "

[67]Mayer I. Gruber, *Aspects of Nonverbal Communication in the Ancient Near East* (Rome: Biblical Institute Press, 1980), 371. For this argument see pp. 357, 371-79.

[68] See, e.g., Walter Brueggemann, "Life and Death in Tenth Century Israel," *Journal of the American Academy of Religion* 40 (1972): 101.

In the syntax of the sentence primary stress falls upon the noun נְבָלָה, object of the verb "to do" (עשׂה). Translating it as "outrage" (NRSV), "folly" (RSV), or "insult" (New Jerusalem Bible),[69] scholars recognized the special meaning of the noun. For example, Gerhard von Rad places the word in the context of sexual violence and suggests: "The word for infamous deed (*nebala*) is an ancient expression for the most serious kind of sexual evil."[70] The phrase does not only occur in texts about sexual violence but also in Joshua 7:15, where Achan takes banned goods and God condemns him for it. For such a context Anthony Philipps proposes a related meaning:

> Nebalah [is] not a term reserved for sexual offenses of a particularly abhor-
> rent kind. Rather *nebalah* is a *general expression for serious disorderly
> and unruly action* resulting in the break up of an existing relationship whether
> between tribes, within the family, in a business arrangement, in marriage or
> with God. This shows its *extreme gravity* and perhaps *explains why the
> word is so rarely used.* It indicates the *end of an existing order* consequent
> upon breach of rules which maintained that order.[71] [stress added]

The noun נבלה expresses societal disorder and upheaval caused by serious transgressions. It describes injustice in social and political relations. Rape belongs in this category, constituting the "end of an existing order" and an act of "utterly disorderly and unruly fashion."[72] The doer of נבלה destroys the community's relationship to God. Only the punishment of the perpetrator can reestablish the relationship. As Sarna explains:

> Hebrew *nebalah* is a powerful term describing offenses of such profound
> abhorrence that they threaten to tear apart the fabric of Israelite society. For

---

[69] The New Jerusalem Bible radically departs from the Hebrew by turning the noun into a verb and giving it the subject Shechem: "When Jacob's sons returned from the countryside and heard the news; the men were outraged and infuriated that Shechem had insulted Israel by sleeping with Jacob's daughter—a thing totally unacceptable."

[70] Gerhard von Rad, *Genesis: A Commentary*, The Old Testament Library, trans. John H. Marks, 3rd rev. ed. (Philadelphia: Westminster Press, 1972), 332. See also Erhard Blum, *Die Komposition der Vätergeschichte*, Wissenschaftliche Monographien zum Alten und Neuen Testament, vol. 57 (Neukirchen-Vluyn: Neukirchener Verlag, 1984), 213; Brueggemann, *Genesis*, 276. For other texts that use this word see Deuteronomy 22:21, Judges 19:23, 2 Samuel 13:12.

[71] Anthony Philipps, "NEBALAH," *Vetus Testamentum* 25 (1975): 241.

[72] Ibid., 238.

society's own self-protection, such atrocities can never be tolerated or left unpunished.[73]

Characterized as נבלה, rape changes the social relations within the community in the following way: Shechem attempted to establish his control over Dinah by raping her. The rape altered Dinah's relationship with her community. The community in turn experienced rape as a disruption of societal harmony. The word נבלה foreshadows the severe response of the brothers toward the perpetrator.[74]

The disorder that Shechem had "done" in Israel is not "done" (עשה). The conclusion of v. 7 plays on the verb עשה. Not referring to a divine law, the last line reports a custom of the people.[75] Israel does not tolerate rape, the narrator claims. The line emphasizes this intolerance by using terminology that relates Dinah's predicament to the broader social setting. The depth of fraternal grief and depression finds support in the clauses "disorder he-did in-Israel" and "so-not it-was-done." The rapist has done what is not done. The positive use of the verb עשה negates the negative.

Reading Scene Two from a feminist standpoint unfolds crucial understandings about rape. Feminist scholarship has pointed out that rape is not only an individual act of sexual violence. It reflects societal, political, and economic conditions of hierarchy and injustice and is symptomatic for societal disorder. As society is implicated in the prevalence of rape, its redress involves society. Feminist scholarship recognizes that the individual treatment of a rapist does not suffice.

Scene Three: The Negotiations (vv. 8-24)
After the fast-moving Scene Two that has jumped from one family to the other, Scene Three brings the families together to negotiate the marriage between Shechem and Dinah. The negotiations proceed uninterrupted. A preponderance of words, including elaborate speeches and frequent repetitions, characterize the scene. Four speeches constitute its major divisions: vv. 8-10, vv. 11-12, vv. 13-17, vv. 18-24.

---

[73] See Sarna, *Genesis*, 234. See also M. Saebo, "נבל nabal," in *Theologisches Handwörterbuch zum Alten Testament*, ed. Ernst Jenni and Claus Westermann, vol. 2 (München: Kaiser, 1976), 26-31; "#1285 נבל (nabal) II, be senseless, foolish," in *Theological Wordbook*, vol. 2, 547f.

[74] Cf. 2 Samuel 13:12.

[75] See, for example, Trible, *Texts of Terror*, 45; Sarna, *Genesis*, 234, 367, footnote 12.

HAMOR (vv. 8-10)

8 And-spoke Hamor to-them the-following: וַיְדַבֵּר חֲמוֹר אִתָּם לֵאמֹר

Shechem my-son, wants his-nepeš your-<u>daughter</u>.   שְׁכֶם בְּנִי חָשְׁקָה נַפְשׁוֹ בְּבִתְּכֶם
Give then her to-him for-a-wife.   תְּנוּ נָא אֹתָהּ לוֹ לְאִשָּׁה׃
9 And-marry with-us,   וְהִתְחַתְּנוּ אֹתָנוּ
your-<u>daughters</u> give to-us   בְּנֹתֵיכֶם תִּתְּנוּ-לָנוּ
and-our-<u>daughters</u> take for-yourselves.   וְאֶת-בְּנֹתֵינוּ תִּקְחוּ לָכֶם׃
10 and-with-us <u>settle</u>,   וְאִתָּנוּ תֵּשֵׁבוּ
and-<u>the-land</u> will-be before-you.   וְהָאָרֶץ תִּהְיֶה לִפְנֵיכֶם
<u>Settle</u>,   שְׁבוּ
move-in-her,   וּסְחָרוּהָ
and-acquire-property in-her.   וְהֵאָחֲזוּ בָּהּ׃

No details inform the reader about Hamor's arrival; yet the negotiations begin with Hamor speaking. Although according to v. 4 he planned to speak only to Jacob, here he addresses both Jacob and his sons, presenting the rationale for the marriage request. The placing of the name "Shechem" with the modifier בְּנִי at the beginning of the sentence functions as an introduction of emphasis. Thereupon comes the verb חשק followed by its subject "his-nepeš." Both in syntax of the sentence and in the context of the story, what Shechem wants is central to who he is: Shechem my-son, wants his-nepeš." Contrary to translations that interpret this verb in the direction of love, its simple meaning is "to want, to take."[76] Accordingly, the Septuagint translates the verb as "προσαιρέομαι." This understanding also correlates with v. 3 where the verb (ב) דבק was not translated as an expression of love but as a reference to spatial closeness: "to remain close."[77] Hamor proposes marriage because Shechem "wants" Dinah as he desires. So Hamor requests: "Give her to-him for-a-wife."

Next Hamor extends the possibilities to propose general intermarriage between the two peoples: "And-marry with-us, your-daughters

---

[76] See, e.g., RSV and NRSV: "longs for;" Jerusalem Bible: "set on;" New English Bible: "is in love."
[77] Hence, the translation of חשק in Gesenius, *Hebräisches Handwörterbuch*, 267, is inappropriate for v. 8. Other examples for the use of this verb appear in Deuteronomy 7:7, 10:15, 21:11, 1 Kings 9:19, Isaiah 38:17, Psalms 91:14, 2 Chronicles 8:6. See also G. Wallis, "חשק ḥašaq," in *Theologisches Wörterbuch zum Alten Testament*, ed. Heinz-Josef Fabry and Helmer Ringgren, vol. 3 (Stuttgart: Kohlhammer, 1982), 280f.

give to-us and-our-daughters take for-yourselves." This idea surprises a reader because Shechem did not mention it in v. 4. If Hamor knows about the rape (cf. v. 6), then perhaps here he is tempting Jacob and his sons to look beyond their immediate concern.

After Hamor invited them to intermarry (v. 9), he then invites them to settle in the land (v. 10). The two invitations are structured similarly. After each general invitation an elaboration of meaning follows. Further, the relationship between the general invitations forms a chiasm: verb and object (v. 9) and object and verb (v. 10).

General Invitation (v. 9)	*General Invitation (v. 10)*
a b	b' a'
And-<u>marry</u> <u>with-us</u>	and-<u>with-us</u> <u>settle</u>
Elaborations	*Elaborations*
your-<u>daughters</u> give to-us	and-the-land will-be before-you.
and-our-<u>daughters</u> take for-yourselves	Settle,
	move-in-her,
	and-acquire-property in-her.

The arrangement of the chiasm has Jacob's family as the subject, encircling Hamor and his people. Attempting to convince them, Hamor pretends that the control lies with Jacob's family. His speech stresses the gains for the Israelites.

Hamor attempts to persuade the family of Jacob to arrange a wedding between Dinah and Shechem, the rapist. The first two lines of his speech present Shechem (v. 8); the remaining verses (vv. 9, 10) present the family with the benefits of accepting this arrangement. They will profit because they will receive women and permanent settlement. The extended elaboration in v. 10 encourages Jacob and his sons to accept the deal. Three imperatives seek to persuade: settle (שׁוּב), move (חסר), and acquire property (אחז). The first verb "settle" repeats the general invitation. To the second and third imperatives are attached feminine suffixes that have as their antecedent "the land" (הארץ). Literally, they read "move in her" and "acquire in her." But Hamor's words carry meanings beyond the surface one. Given the subject of the story, these feminine suffixes subtly allude to Dinah. Shechem "wants" (חשׁק) to "move in her" and "acquire property in her." As Shechem acquired Dinah, so Jacob and his sons should acquire the land. Hamor considers Dinah a bargaining chip. Controlled by men, Dinah is object and property of male discourse. Feminist analysis of rape culture exposed such discourse for its violent implications.

SHECHEM (vv. 11-12)

Another speech is made to tempt the family of Jacob. Hamor did not go alone to negotiate the terms. Shechem accompanied him. After his father's speech Shechem addresses Jacob and his sons.

11 Then-said Shechem to her-father	וַיֹּאמֶר שְׁכֶם אֶל־אָבִיהָ
and-to her-brothers:	וְאֶל־אַחֶיהָ
Let-me-find favor in-your-eyes,	אֶמְצָא־חֵן בְּעֵינֵיכֶם
And-whatever you-say to-me	וַאֲשֶׁר תֹּאמְרוּ אֵלַי
I-will-give.	אֶתֵּן׃
12 Raise for-me much bride-price and-present,	הַרְבּוּ עָלַי מְאֹד מֹהַר וּמַתָּן
and-let-me-give,	וְאֶתְּנָה
whatever you-say to-me,	כַּאֲשֶׁר תֹּאמְרוּ אֵלָי
but-give to-me the-young-woman for-a-wife.	וּתְנוּ־לִי אֶת־הַנַּעֲרָ לְאִשָּׁה׃

Repetition of vocabulary and of grammatical forms secures the major sections. Similarity of themes then falls into place. The speech is arranged in a chiasm:

A <u>Let-me-find favor in-your-eyes,</u>
B <u>and-whatever you-say to-me</u>
C <u>I-will-give.</u>
D *Raise for-me much bride-price and-present,*
C' and-let-me-give,
B' <u>Whatever you-say to-me</u>
A' <u>but-give to-me the-young-woman for-a-wife.</u>

As the beginning and end of the units, A and A' are joined by similar verbal constructions and by similarity of theme. Both contain imperatives: A begins with a cohortative and A' with an imperative of second person plural. In A Shechem seeks a favor; in A' the favor is specified. B and B' are virtually identical. Each begins with the partical אֲשֶׁר. Using deferential speech with Jacob and his sons as subjects, Shechem seeks to get what he wants. The deference continues in C and C' where Shechem himself is the subject: "I-will-give . . . and-let-me-give." His first person speech surrounds the second person imperative (pl.) to ensnare with a generous offer. This offer is the center of the chiasm: "Raise for-me much bride-price and-present." Pretended hu-

mility and modesty characterize Shechem's speech. However, the brothers cannot give Dinah because Shechem has already taken her to his
house without either their permission or hers. He is the giver and
fulfiller of his request. Feminist scholarship teaches that after the rape
the rapist can often appear in good presence.

THE BROTHERS (vv. 13-17)

In this section the sons of Jacob answer Shechem and his father Hamor.
Their speech shows its centrality in several ways. It constitutes the
middle of the thirty-one verses. Three speeches precede, and three
follow it. The family relations of son (A) and father (B) serve as the
organizing principle:

A	Speech 1	son:	Shechem	(v. 4)
B	Speech 2	father:	Hamor	(vv. 8-10)
A	Speech 3	son:	Shechem	(vv. 11-12)
A	Speech 4	sons:	Jacob's sons	(vv. 14-17)
AB	Speech 5	son and father:	Shechem and Hamor	(vv. 21-23)
B	Speech 6	father:	Jacob	(v. 30)
A	Speech 7	sons:	Jacob's sons	(v. 31)

As the center of Genesis 34 the speech by Jacob's sons (Speech 4)
is significant for the development of the story. The brothers pretend to
negotiate with the rapist and his father, but the narrated introduction
(v. 13) to their speech discloses their real motivation. Three times the
narrator introduces their speech: "they answered . . . they spoke . . .
they said" (וַיֵּעֲנוּ ;וַיְדַבֵּרוּ ;וַיֹּאמְרוּ).

Verses 13-14a

13　Then-answered the-sons-of Jacob to-Shechem　　　　　　　וַיַּעֲנוּ בְנֵי־יַעֲקֹב אֶת־שְׁכֶם
　　　and-to-Hamor, his-father, with-cleverness　　　　　　　וְאֶת־חֲמוֹר אָבִיו בְּמִרְמָה
　　　and-they-spoke　　　　　　　　　　　　　　　　　　　　　וַיְדַבֵּרוּ
　　　　　　because he-had-oppressed Dinah, their sister.　אֲשֶׁר טִמֵּא אֵת דִּינָה אֲחֹתָם׃
14a　And-they-said to-them:　　　　　　　　　　　　　　　　וַיֹּאמְרוּ אֲלֵיהֶם

The first verb is fascinating because its root is ענה, the same root
used in v. 2 rendered as "to rape." Here in v. 13 the verb is in the qal
and means "to answer." In repeating the verbal stem the narrator indicates that the brothers do not forget the reason for the negotiation.

Always aware of the rape, they do not get trapped by the many words
of Hamor and Shechem. They negotiate because of the rape, and they
negotiate with cleverness. The noun מִרְמָה suggests that the brothers
make a proposal without arousing suspicion about their real intent. As
Jacob once resorted to trickery to obtain a blessing (Genesis 27), now
his sons use "cleverness" to outwit the rapist. The Jewish medieval
interpreter Rashi writes: "You think this is trickery! Not at all! . . .
Trickery is justified when it is a matter of a punishment for an immoral
act as disgusting as this one."[78]

The brothers move at a slow pace; it takes three starts to give the
right response. First they answer, second they speak. Following this
verb comes the motivation for their speech, Shechem's rape of their
sister Dinah. As in v. 5, טמא refers to the rape as an act of communal
disorder. The third verb "to say" leads directly to their speech.

The speech divides into two main sections. The first opens with the
particle לֹא (v. 14b) and concludes with a כִּי-clause (v. 14e). The second opens with the particle אַךְ, introducing a general statement about
the forthcoming agreement: "Only for-this we-will-agree with-you" (v.
15a). Following this general statement come two subsections, each
introduced by the particle אִם. The first gives the positive side of the
agreement: "if" (v. 15b-16). The second gives the negative: "if not" (v.
17).

Verses 14b-17

14b Not (לֹא) we-can do the-thing the-this   לֹא נוּכַל לַעֲשׂוֹת הַדָּבָר הַזֶּה
    to-give our-sister to-a-man   לָתֵת אֶת־אֲחֹתֵנוּ לְאִישׁ
    who to-him (is) a-foreskin   אֲשֶׁר־לוֹ עָרְלָה
    because (כִּי) a-disgrace he-is for-us.   כִּי־חֶרְפָּה הִוא לָנוּ׃

---

[78] For other noncontemporary Jewish interpretations see Eli Munk, *The Call of
the Torah: An Anthology of Interpretation and Commentary of the Five Books
of Moses*, transl. E. S. Mazer (New York: Mesorah, 1994), 462.

[79] The Masoretic pointing suggests to read the personal pronoun as the third
person feminine "she," referring to the feminine nouns "foreskin" or "disgrace." The
consonants of the pronoun (scriptio plena), however, suggest the masculine pronoun
"he," referring to the noun "a man." The ambiguity of the present Hebrew text
shows that both pronouns are possible and make sense. The Masoretic vocalization,
however, smoothed away the reference to Shechem by diverting the attention from
Shechem to the foreskin. Since the "uncircumcised *man*" is the problem and not the
"foreskin" per se, the scriptio plena is preferable.

15 *Only (אַךְ) for-this we-will-agree with-you:*   אַךְ־בְּזֹאת נֵאוֹת לָכֶם

    If (אִם) you-become like-us   אִם תִּהְיוּ כָמֹנוּ

        to-circumcise from-you every male.   לְהִמֹּל לָכֶם כָּל־זָכָר:

16 *Then-we-will-give our-daughters to-you*   וְנָתַנוּ אֶת־בְּנֹתֵינוּ לָכֶם

    and-your-daughters we-will-take for-us.   וְאֶת־בְּנֹתֵיכֶם נִקַּח־לָנוּ

    Then we-will-settle with-you   וְיָשַׁבְנוּ אִתְּכֶם

    and-we-will-be one people.   וְהָיִינוּ לְעַם אֶחָד:

17 *But-if not (אִם־לֹא) you-hear to-us*   וְאִם־לֹא תִשְׁמְעוּ אֵלֵינוּ

    to circumcise,   לְהִמֹּל

    then-we-will-take our- daughter   וְלָקַחְנוּ אֶת־בִּתֵּנוּ

    and-we-will-go.   וְהָלָכְנוּ:

Characterized by verbs in the first person plural, the speech of the brothers explains the conditions for marriage. The first sentence, "Not we-can do (לַעֲשׂוֹת) this thing" (v. 14), alludes to v. 7, where the root עשׂה was used twice: "because disorder he-did (עשׂה) in Israel to-lay the-daughter-of Jacob and-so not it-was-done (יֵעָשֶׂה)." For the third time the root appears and connects to the second time it was used: "and-so not it-was-done" (v. 7g). Now the brothers admit, "Not we-can do the-thing the-this" (V. 14b). Only the next line explains that this time the phrase does not allude to the rape. The following phrase introduced by an infinitive refers to marriage. The verb of the infinitive "to give (נתן)" recapitulates the vocabulary of Hamor's (v. 8) and Shechem's speech (v. 11, 12). Now the brothers specify a reason for their refusal to give: that Shechem is uncircumcised.

Their proposal features two possibilities. The first is the acceptance of circumcision, which would lead to intermarriage (v. 15) and to settlement (v. 16), indeed, to becoming "one people" (v. 16d). The second is the rejection of circumcision, which would result in their "taking (לקח)" Dinah back (v. 17). At this point an important detail emerges: Dinah is already at the house of Shechem. Thus, Jacob's family does not have the liberty to reject outright the offer by Hamor and Shechem because Dinah is with them. So the brothers pretend to play along with Dinah's kidnapper. But they set up conditions for accepting. They propose circumcision.

HAMOR AND SHECHEM (vv. 18-24)

In the final speech of Scene Three, Hamor and Shechem address their townspeople. Preceding this speech, narrated discourse reports their own reaction to the speech of the brothers.

Verses 18-20

18 And-good-appeared their-words   וַיִּיטְבוּ דִבְרֵיהֶם בְּעֵינֵי חֲמוֹר וּבְעֵינֵי שְׁכֶם
    in-the-eyes-of Hamor and-in-the-eyes-of Shechem
                  the-son-of Hamor.   בֶּן־חֲמוֹר:

19 So-not waited the-young-man   וְלֹא־אֵחַר הַנַּעַר
    to-do the-thing   לַעֲשׂוֹת הַדָּבָר
    because (כִּי) he-desired the-daughter-of Jacob   כִּי חָפֵץ בְּבַת־יַעֲקֹב
    and-he-was the-most-powerful in-the-whole house-of   וְהוּא נִכְבָּד מִכֹּל בֵּית אָבִיו:
    his-father.

20 And-came Hamor and-Shechem, his son, to   וַיָּבֹא חֲמוֹר וּשְׁכֶם בְּנוֹ אֶל־שַׁעַר עִירָם
    the-gate-of their-town,
    and-they-spoke to the-people-of their-town: וַיְדַבְּרוּ אֶל־אַנְשֵׁי עִירָם לֵאמֹר:

Hamor and Shechem like what they have heard. Once again the
story plays on the verb עשׂה (cf. vv. 7,14). The report suggests that
the townspeople comply because of Shechem's high position as "the-
most-powerful in-the-whole house-of his-father" (v. 19d).

Within the narrated discourse appears one remarkable rhetorical
device. The particle כִּי in v. 19 presents the reason why Shechem
accepted the conditions of Dinah's brothers so quickly: "because (כִּי)
he-desired (חפץ) the-daughter-of Jacob." G. Gerleman comments that
the erb חפץ often expresses "the favor of a legally or socially higher
standing person to a person somehow dependent on him."[80] The verb
plays on social class differences. G. J. Botterweck proposes to translate חפץ as "to want, to lust for, to desire."[81] Similar to the translation
of חשׁק (to want, v. 8), אהב (to lust after, v. 3), and דבק (ב) (to remain
close, v. 3), the verb חפץ does not regard the response of the other
person. Shechem has accepted the conditions because he wants to get
his chosen object. Different Hebrew verbs express the fact that his
desire to continue the dynamics of rape dominates his activity. His
father complies.

---

[80] G. Gerleman, "חפץ ḥpṣ," in *Theologisches Handwörterbuch zum Alten Testament*, ed. Ernst Jenni and Claus Westermann, vol. 1 (München: Kaiser, 1971),
624: "die Gunst eines rechtlich oder gesellschaftlich Höherherstehenden zu einem
von ihm irgendwie Abhängigen." Gerleman does not place Genesis 34:19 in this
category but assumes that Shechem loved Dinah. He disregards the power difference
between Dinah and Shechem.

[81] G. J. Botterweck, "חפץ ḥāpēṣ," in *Theologisches Wörterbuch zum Alten
Testament*, ed. Heinz-Josef Fabry and Helmer Ringgren, vol. 3 (Stuttgart:
Kohlhammer, 1982), 102, 108.

Verse 21

21 The-people the-these <u>are-peaceful</u> they with-us.   הָאֲנָשִׁים הָאֵלֶּה שְׁלֵמִים הֵם אִתָּנוּ
    <u>They-will-settle in-the-land</u>   וְיֵשְׁבוּ בָאָרֶץ
    and-they-will-trade her   וְיִסְחֲרוּ אֹתָהּ
    and-<u>the-land</u>, behold (הִנֵּה) , width-of hands before-them וְהָאָרֶץ הִנֵּה רַחֲבַת־יָדַיִם לִפְנֵיהֶם
    them.
    Their-**daughters** we-will-take for-us for wives   אֶת־בְּנֹתָם נִקַּח־לָנוּ לְנָשִׁים
    And-our-**daughters** we-will-give to-them.   וְאֶת־בְּנֹתֵינוּ נִתֵּן לָהֶם׃

Father and son now speak directly to the people of their town. The arrangement of the speech shows rhetorical skills. The unit has two sections. In the first section they present the benefits of their proposal: "The-people the-these are-peaceful they with-us" (v. 21). The speech begins with a word new to the discourse: peaceful (שְׁלֵמִים). It gives a favorable characterization of the Israelites. The section continues in two subsections that use earlier vocabulary. The first subsection pertains to the land (cf. v. 10), and it draws upon the earlier vocabulary of Hamor's speech (vv. 8-10): "settle," "trade," and "before you/ them." The last line reinforces the earlier speech by the inclusion of the particle הִנֵּה and the more elaborate description of the land ("thewidth-of hands before-them," cf. v. 10). The second subsection pertains to the "daughters" (v. 21d, e). For the third time in the story the issue of intermarriage arises (cf. 9, 16).

A comparison of the three occurrences shows significant differences in the word order and the subjects of the verbs, thereby disclosing the ulterior motive behind Hamor's offer. In v. 9 Hamor invites Jacob and his sons:

<u>Your-daughters</u> <u>give</u> <u>to-us</u>   בְּנֹתֵיכֶם תִּתְּנוּ־לָנוּ
And-<u>our-daughters</u> take **for-yourselves.**   אֶת־בְּנֹתֵינוּ תִּקְחוּ לָכֶם׃

In v. 16 the brothers answer:

Then-<u>we-will-give</u> <u>our-daughters</u> **to-you**   וְנָתַנּוּ אֶת־בְּנֹתֵינוּ לָכֶם
And-<u>your-daughters</u> we-will-take <u>for-us.</u>   וְאֶת־בְּנֹתֵיכֶם נִקַּח־לָנוּ

Here in v. 21 Shechem and Hamor say to their townspeople:

Their-<u>daughters</u> we-will-take <u>for-us</u> as-wives   אֶת־בְּנֹתָם נִקַּח־לָנוּ לְנָשִׁים
And-<u>our-daughters</u> <u>we-will-give</u> to-them.   וְאֶת־בְּנֹתֵינוּ נִתֵּן לָהֶם׃

Parallelism organizes the first occurrence. Coming first in the sentence, the object "daughters" precedes the verbs in the plural imperative which is then followed by the pronoun לְ. In attempting to hide their real motives for the marriage proposal, Hamor and Shechem give the daughters primary emphasis. By contrast, in the second occurrence the verbs in the first person plural enclose the object "daughters." The order of the words indicates that the brothers protect the daughters, including Dinah. The third occurrence is similar to the first. Again the object "daughters" precedes the verbs in the plural imperative, followed by the pronoun. But the grammatical reversal of verbs and person signals a reversal of power. In the first occurrence Jacob's family is invited to be the agent of action. In the third the Shechemites themselves are the agents. Good marketing is used to convince the people.

The different goals of the brothers and of Hamor and Shechem become pronounced in regard to two other details. In the second occurrence the brothers begin with "our" daughters and only then refer to "your" daughters. They pretend generosity by giving their women first. In the first and third occurrence this order is reversed. Hamor and Shechem refer first to "your" and "their" daughters and then to "our" daughters. They request that the brothers give their daughters before Hamor and Shechem give theirs. Hamor and Shechem take before they give, a subtle point that uncovers their real motives.

An inclusion delineates the second section. It begins and ends with the particle אַךְ, with the verb "to agree" (אות), and with the verb "to settle" (ישׁב).

Verses 22-23

22 Only (אַךְ) for-this will-agree <u>with-us</u> the-men   אַךְ־בְּזֹאת יֵאֹתוּ לָנוּ הָאֲנָשִׁים
      to-settle <u>with-us</u>   לָשֶׁבֶת אִתָּנוּ
      to-be people one: לִהְיוֹת לְעַם אֶחָד
      to-circumcise <u>for-us</u> all males,   בְּהִמּוֹל לָנוּ כָּל־זָכָר
      as they are-circumcised.   כַּאֲשֶׁר הֵם נִמֹּלִים׃
23 Their-livestock and-their-property and-all-of their-   מִקְנֵהֶם וְקִנְיָנָם וְכָל־בְּהֶמְתָּם
      animals,
      shall-not (be) <u>for-us</u> they?   הֲלוֹא לָנוּ הֵם
      Only (אַךְ) let-us-agree with-them   אַךְ נֵאוֹתָה לָהֶם
      and-<u>they-will-settle</u> <u>with-us.</u>   וְיֵשְׁבוּ אִתָּנוּ׃

Within the inclusio first comes familiar vocabulary and themes: "to be one people" (cf. 16) and male circumcision (cf. v. 15). The familiar is followed by new content: the promise of possessing their livestock and their property. As the section unfolds, the requirement of circumcision is tucked between two attractive possibilities. Indeed, the reference to circumcision does not even contain an inflected verb but an infinitive and a participle: בְּהִמֹּל‎and מֻלִים‎. In their speech the ultimate gain rests with the townspeople. If they agree, they will own the livestock, property, and animals. The master of marketing, Hamor, ends on a tempting note: "Will not their livestock, their property, and all their animals be ours?" (NRSV). Similar to Hamor's first speech (vv. 8-10), the addressees are the grammatical subject, and thus have the illusion of authority. However, the emphasis on the gain for those who are addressed conceals Hamor's and Shechem's real motive.

After their speech indirect discourse reports the circumcision. The ominous deed is described with three brief words: "And-was-circumcised every male." The parallel clauses surrounding the act emphasize its inclusivity: "all those-going-out to-the-gate-of his-town."

Verse 24

24 So-heard to-Hamor and-to-Shechem, his son,	וַיִּשְׁמְעוּ אֶל־חֲמוֹר וְאֶל־שְׁכֶם בְּנוֹ
all those-going-out to-the-gate-of his-town.	כָּל־יֹצְאֵי שַׁעַר עִירוֹ
And-was-circumcised every male	וַיִּמֹּלוּ כָּל־זָכָר
all those-going-out to-the-gate-of his-town.	כָּל־יֹצְאֵי שַׁעַר עִירוֹ:

Scene Four: The Killing (vv. 25-29)

The time for speeches is over. The brothers prepare the revenge. They kill not only the rapist and his father but all the males of the town. On the one hand, the brothers recognize rape not only as a problem between two individuals but as a crime with societal dimension. They demonstrate with their action that the entire town, as a societal entity, participates in rape and rape-prone behavior. Everybody is involved, not only Shechem, the rapist. On the other hand, the brothers treat the women and children of the town as they did not like their sister to be treated. They not only take them—in fact, they capture them. Differentiating between "our" and "their" women, the brothers engage in a patriarchal mode of thinking and acting. As characters of this story, Dinah's brothers personify the contradictory approach toward sexual violence that defends one's "own" woman at the expense of other women.

SIMEON AND LEVI (vv. 25-26)

Two sections of narrated discourse (vv. 25-26 and vv. 27-29) present the measure undertaken by the brothers. In the first the brothers Simeon and Levi take the lead.

Verses 25-26

25 Then on-the-day the-third,	וַיְהִי בַיּוֹם הַשְּׁלִישִׁי
when-they-felt pains,	בִּהְיוֹתָם כֹּאֲבִים
and-<u>took</u> the-two sons-of Jacob, Simeon and-Levi,	וַיִּקְחוּ שְׁנֵי־בְנֵי־יַעֲקֹב שִׁמְעוֹן וְלֵוִי
the-brothers-of Dinah, each his-sword.	אֲחֵי דִינָה אִישׁ חַרְבּוֹ
They-came to-the-town unaware	וַיָּבֹאוּ עַל־הָעִיר בֶּטַח
And-<u>they-killed</u> every male.	וַיַּהַרְגוּ כָּל־זָכָר׃
26 And-Hamor and-Shechem, his-son,	וְאֶת־חֲמוֹר וְאֶת־שְׁכֶם בְּנוֹ
<u>they-killed</u> with the-sword	הָרְגוּ לְפִי־חָרֶב
and-<u>they-took</u> Dinah from-the-house-of Shechem	וַיִּקְחוּ אֶת־דִּינָה מִבֵּית שְׁכֶם
and-<u>they-went-out</u>.	וַיֵּצֵאוּ׃

The importance of the third day (v. 25) appears in many biblical texts. It represents a segment of time after which new and decisive events follow a previous event. On the third day people are ready for the new action. For example, on the third day Laban hears that Jacob has fled (Genesis 31:22). On the third day, when Pharaoh celebrates his birthday, he restores the chief cupbearer and kills the baker (Genesis 40:20). On the third day all the tribes of Israel gather against the Benjaminites to punish them for their wrongdoing against the concubine of the Levite (Judges 20:30).[82] The third day constitutes then "a significant segment of time" in biblical storytelling.[83] The appropriate period of time in which "to prepare important things,"[84] three days include the reflection on the past on the first day, the preparation and evaluation of the plan on the second day, and the new action on the third day.[85]

---

[82] For further references see Genesis 42:18; Leviticus 7:17,18;19:6,7; Numbers 7:24; 19:12,19; 29:20; 31:19; Joshua 9:17; 1 Samuel 30:1; 2 Samuel 1:2.

[83] Nahum M. Sarna, *Exodus*, The JPS Torah Commentary (Philadelphia: Jewish Publication Society, 1991), 105, on Exodus 19:11: "Prepare for the third day, because on the third day YHWH will come down upon Mount Sinai in the sight of all the people."

[84] Jacob, *Genesis*, 495, on Genesis 22:4: "On the third day Abraham looked up and saw the place far away."

[85] Ibid.: "Am ersten Tage steckt man noch im Alten, am dritten tritt man in das Neue, der zweite ist ausschließlich Vorbereitung und Erwartung."

During three days the brothers had time to consider their intention and to prepare the next step. The reference to the third day indicates that they did not act in a compulsive, blind, and hurried way but in a deliberate, calculated, and concise one.

Typical of biblical narrative, the significance of the number three is apparent elsewhere in Genesis 34. Often three verbs structure the action. In v. 2 and v. 3, three verbs describe the rape and three de-scribe Shechem's control over Dinah. The verbal root טמא occurs three times (vv. 5, 13, and 27). Three times someone "goes out" (יצא, vv. 1, 6, and 26). In v. 10 three imperatives end Hamor's speech: "Settle, move-in-her, and-acquire-property in-her." The brothers start three times to respond to the proposals of Hamor and Shechem (vv. 13 and 14). In addition to verbal repetition three parts structure the fraternal response in v. 7 and three times the intermarriage proposal is given (vv. 9, 16, 21). The rhetorical structure of the narrative highlights the revenge on the third day by playing on the theme of "three" through-out the narrative.

Verses 25-26 describe the vengeful killing by Simeon and Levi, characterized as "brothers-of Dinah." Two sets of three verbs each structure the action:

a	take (לקח)	c'	kill (חרג)
b	come (בוא)	a'	take (לקח)
c	kill (חרג)	d	go out (יצא)

The verb "to kill" (חרג) ends the first set and begins the second, thereby surrounding the objects "every male" and "Hamor and Shechem, his son." Form and content make it impossible to escape the attack. The verb לקח appears also twice, combined with "sword" (v. 25) and with "Dinah" (v. 26), as if to say that only the sword has made possible the liberation of Dinah from the house of Shechem. The two remaining verbs are opposites: to come (בוא) and to go (יצא). The verb יצא is last in the series. After the bloodshed the brothers leave. This verb appears three times: Dinah goes out (v. 1), Hamor leaves to negotiate with Jacob (v. 6), and Dinah and her brothers go out from the house of the killed rapist (v. 26).

THE BROTHERS (vv. 27-29)

In the second section of this scene, the other brothers, who are not named, continue the revenge begun by Simeon and Levi. They plun-der the town and take women and children as captives. Now another group of men threatens the women and children of the man who raped their sister. Defending Dinah, the brothers do not extend their defense to other women.

27 The-sons-of Jacob came to the-killed-men	בְּנֵי יַעֲקֹב בָּאוּ עַל־הַחֲלָלִים
and-they-<u>plundered</u> the-town	וַיָּבֹזּוּ הָעִיר
because they-had-oppressed their-sister.	אֲשֶׁר טִמְּאוּ אֲחוֹתָם:
28 Their-flocks	אֶת־צֹאנָם
and-their-herds	וְאֶת־בְּקָרָם
and-their-donkeys	וְאֶת־חֲמֹרֵיהֶם
and-that in-his-town	וְאֵת אֲשֶׁר־בָּעִיר
and-<u>that</u> in-the-field	וְאֶת־אֲשֶׁר בַּשָּׂדֶה
they-took.	לָקָחוּ:
29 And <u>all</u> their-wealth	וְאֶת־כָּל־חֵילָם
and <u>all</u> their-babies	וְאֶת־כָּל־טַפָּם
and-their-women	וְאֶת־נְשֵׁיהֶם
they-captured	שָׁבוּ
and-they-<u>plundered</u>	וַיָּבֹזּוּ
and <u>all</u> <u>that</u> in-the-house.	וְאֵת כָּל־אֲשֶׁר בַּבָּיִת:

For the third time emphasis is placed on the rape as the controlling event: "because they-had oppressed their-sister" (cf. vv. 5 and 13). For the third time the verb טמא appears; here explaining the fraternal plunder. Remarkably, the verb is in the third person plural; the whole town, not only Shechem the rapist, "oppressed" Dinah. The rape of the sister remains the motive for their brutal and violent action, and so the revenge is directed toward the whole town. Feminist scholarship on rape has recognized that rape not only reflects the action of the rapist but constitutes a societal structural problem. The violence with which the brothers avenge the rape of their sister indicates this understanding. At the same time their action shows their prejudiced view on women. Structural observations illustrate this point.

The verb "to plunder" (בזז) surrounds the description of the seized items, "women" are among them. The items come in sets of three. The first and third sets appear in sequence: "their-flocks and-their-herds and-their donkeys" and "all their-wealth and all their-babies and their-women." Structurally, the second set is incomplete.

The lines are arranged in pairs of three, but the second of the three lines is incomplete. After "that in-his-town" and "that in-the-fields" a third item would be expected, but it is missing. The phrase "all that in-the-house" is this third item, placed at the very end of the unit. It

---

[86] Cf. Trible, *Rhetorical Criticism*, 222, for "the strategy of delayed information."

1.	2.	3.
They-plundered the town,		
1. their-flocks	and-their-herds	and-their-donkeys
2. and-that in-his-town	and-that in-the-fields	_____
they took,		
3. all their-wealth	and all their-babies	and _____ their-women
they captured		
and they plundered		
and all that in-the-house.		

completes the description of the three items in the second pair.[86] The
structure with the final stress on Shechem's house invites the interpretation that "all" happens because of Shechem's house. This unit
accents Shechem's house, to which Dinah was brought. Several verses
earlier Simeon and Levi took Dinah from "the house of Shechem" (v.
26). The phrase "all that in-the-house" refers to this particular house
and is therefore central to the plundering.

   This last phrase "and all that in-the-house" includes the word "all"
(כָּל) which is missing in the third line: "all their-wealth, and-all their-
babies, and _____ their-women." The switch from the third item in the
third line to the final phrase also emphasizes Shechem's house. The
brothers plunder the whole town and all, especially "all that (is)" in the
house of Shechem. The rape affects the whole population. Men are
killed, material goods are taken away, and women and children are
taken captive. The narrated discourse lists children and women as the
last part of the property, maybe as the most valuable. The brothers
capture them because they commit revenge on the enemy men. The
fight is between the men; children, women, and the rest of the property serve merely as the props. Although the brothers respond so
sincerely when they hear about the rape in v. 7, they do not expand
their worry to include the women of their enemies. Staying in a mindset
that differentiates between "our" and "their" women, the brothers
defend only Dinah. In this regard, the story illustrates also the serious
contradictions that men may feel in their responses to rape.

   The verses invite yet another thought. Feminist scholarship emphasizes that society supports rape. Institutions, media, churches, and
even jokes strengthen rape-prone behavior. The extent of the fraternal revenge recognizes the problem of societal participation. The brothers do not confine their anger to the rapist. They avenge the rape by
punishing everybody, killing men and capturing women and children.

Everybody is implicated in the oppressive and violent behavior of rape—
a radical idea. The literary structure of vv. 27-29 underlines that plunder assaults the whole city because of the actions of Shechem, the
rapist.

Scene Five: Jacob and Simeon and Levi (vv. 30-31)

The revenge is complete. Dinah is back. Her brothers have returned,
bringing with her the captives. Seeing what has happened, Jacob the
father finally speaks. He condemns Simeon and Levi for their deed.

Verse 30

30 Said Jacob to Simeon and-to Levi:

וַיֹּאמֶר יַעֲקֹב אֶל־שִׁמְעוֹן וְאֶל־לֵוִי

You-brought-trouble to-me	עֲכַרְתֶּם אֹתִי
to-make-me-odious among-the-settlers-of-the-land,	לְהַבְאִישֵׁנִי בְּיֹשֵׁב הָאָרֶץ
among-the-Canaanites and-the Perizzites.	בַּכְּנַעֲנִי וּבַפְּרִזִּי
And-I am-small in-number	וַאֲנִי מְתֵי מִסְפָּר
and-they-will-gather against-me	וְנֶאֶסְפוּ עָלַי
and-they-attack-me,	וְהִכּוּנִי
and-I-will-be-destroyed,	וְנִשְׁמַדְתִּי
I and-my-house.	אֲנִי וּבֵיתִי

Jacob focuses on the trouble their deeds bring to him and his house.
Rhetorically, first person pronouns dominate his speech: "You-brought-
trouble to-*me*, to-make-*me*-odious among-the settlers-of-the-land, . . .
I-*am*-small in-number, and-they-will-gather against-*me* and-they-attack-
me, and-I-*will*-be-destroyed, I and-*my*-house." The pronoun אֲנִי surrounds three verbs: "to gather," "to attack," and "to destroy." Jacob is
the center of his own attention. He opposes not the rapist but his
sons, though he does not accuse them of being killers and plunderers.
Not the rape, not the killing, not the plunder, and not even his daughter Dinah but his own situation causes him worry.

The final word in the narrative, however, does not belong to Jacob
but to Simeon and Levi. Rather than answering the self-concerned
complaint of their father, they emphasize their sister and her well-
being. They respond with a rhetorical question.

Verse 31

31 And-they-said:

וַיֹּאמְרוּ

Like-a-prostitute he-makes our-sister.	הַכְזוֹנָה יַעֲשֶׂה אֶת־אֲחוֹתֵנוּ

Interpreters sometimes wondered why the brothers refer here to prostitution. Some considered the verse a later addition and thus not relevant for discussions on prostitution in ancient Israel. For instance, Hannelis Schulte considers v. 31 as an addition. She proposes that the term זונה (prostitute) had different meanings in different periods. In early narratives, preceding the monarchic period, the term does not refer to prostitutes but to women who lived within matrilinear family structures. Only when patriarchy and patrilinearity gained dominance, the noun meant "prostitute."[87] Not discussing v. 31, other scholars explain the general situation of Israelite prostitutes. Phyllis A. Bird maintains that financial need forced women to prostitute themselves. As a prostitute, a woman was an outcast and a "dishonored member of society."[88]

The reference to Dinah as a prostitute in v. 31 makes sense when prostitution is understood as a means to financial gain. The brothers refused to sell Dinah into marriage because they did not seek economic gain from the rape. Shechem offered a sum of money, the מֹהַר which was a customary price to get a bride, and assumed that he fulfilled his obligations as a bridegroom.[89] The brothers, however, did not isolate the marriage offer from the rape. They understood that Shechem sought to pay for his deed and called his payment euphemistically מֹהַר. The brothers saw through Shechem's attempt to turn rape into paid sex. They insisted that Dinah was not a prostitute who offered sexual favors and then received payment.[90] They questioned that

---

[87] Hannelis Schulte, "Beobachtungen zum Begriff der Zona im Alten Testament," *Zeitschrift für die alttestamentliche Wissenschaft* 104 (1992): 255-62. Since she regards v. 31 as secondary, Genesis 34 does not oppose her reconstruction of Israelite prostitution, see ibid., p. 257.

[88] Bird, "Harlot as Heroine," 120. For a similar understanding of prostitution in ancient Israel see Renate Jost, "Von 'Huren und Heiligen': Ein sozialgeschichtlicher Beitrag," in *Feministische Hermeneutik und Erstes Testament*, ed. Hedwig Jahnow a. o. (Stuttgart: Kohlhammer, 1994), 126-37. See also the brief remarks on prostitution in relation to 1 Kings 3:16-28 by Gina Hens-Piazza, *Of Methods, Monarchs, and Meanings: A Sociorhetorical Approach to Exegesis* (Macon, GA: Mercer University Press, 1996), 132-34.

[89] Roland de Vaux, *Ancient Israel: Its Life and Institutions* (London: Darton, 1961), 26. Describing Israelite marriage customs, he points out that the noun מֹהַר appears only three times in the Bible (Genesis 34:12; Exodus 22:16; 1 Samuel 18:25). He cautions whether a bridegroom "really" bought the bride.

[90] For the reconstruction of prostitution in ancient Israel see Phyllis A. Bird, "The Harlot as Heroine: Narrative Art and Social Presupposition in Three Old Testament Texts," *Semeia* 46 (1989): 120.

the payment was like a מֹהַר because it was given after a rape. Not in need of financial gain, the brothers rejected the possibility that Shechem would repair his deed through payment. Dinah could not be bought like prostitutes in ancient Israel who needed economic support.[91]

The brothers criticized their father because he failed to acknowledge the ulterior motive behind Hamor and Shechem's marriage proposal. Hiding the rape, Hamor and Shechem promised the family of Dinah economic gain as the central reason for marriage. Hamor said: "With-us settle, and-the-land will-be before-you. Settle, move-in-her, and-acquire-property in-her" (v. 10). Shechem proposed: "Raise for-me much bride-price and-present" (v. 12). Hamor and Shechem believed that money would buy them Dinah, even after the rape. Dinah's brothers, however, followed a different model in which their sister cannot be traded for economic gain. Like the first words in the story ("and-went-out Dinah . . . our-sister"), the last focus on Dinah ("like-a-prostitute he-makes our-sister"). Ending with a question, Genesis 34 calls for an answer beyond this story.

Summary

Open-ended in design, Genesis 34 has attracted various interpretive approaches and perspectives. Here a feminist perspective guided the interpretation that accentuated the rape and presented the chapter as Dinah's story. Since it cannot be assumed that the events of Genesis 34 ever happened,[92] the interpretation presented in this chapter illuminated literary features and highlighted Dinah as the key figure.

Four basic assumptions undergird this chapter. First, the rape is the central concern for this reading. All the other events happen as a consequence of it. As feminist scholarship has raised rape to a promi-

---

[91] Elaine Adler Goodfriend, "Prostitution, Old Testament," *The Anchor Bible Dictionary*, vol. 5 (1992), 505-10; Phyllis A. Bird, "'To Play the Harlot': An Inquiry into an Old Testament Metaphor," in *Gender and Difference in Ancient Israel*, ed. Peggy L. Day (Minneapolis: Fortress, 1989), 75-94. For a contemporary feminist disussion of prostitution see Elizabeth M. Bounds, "Sexuality and Economic Reality: A First World and Third World Comparison," in *Redefining Sexual Ethics: A Sourcebook of Essays, Stories, and Poems*, ed. Susan E. Davies and Eleanor H. Haney (Cleveland: Pilgrim Press, 1991), 131-43; Thanh-dam Truong, *Sex, Money, and Morality: Prostitution and Tourism in South-East Asia* (London: Zed Books, 1990).

[92] For the sometimes contradictory debate about the historical issues involved in Genesis 34 see chapter 2.

nent issue, so the rape is the reason for telling the story of Genesis 34.

Second, rape must be understood from the perspective of the victim-survivor. Thus, this chapter reads Genesis 34 as a story about Dinah. The task was difficult because Dinah never speaks. The literary analysis showed, however, that despite this silence Dinah is present throughout the story. Indeed, everything happens because of her. Informed by feminist scholarship, the reading does not even require her explicit comments. It is clear that she does not like to be raped. Not one feminist study shows that women approve of marrying their rapists. Feminist scholars and activists reject such a practice.[93] Reading Genesis 34 from the perspective of Dinah, an exegete discovers that the story does not present simple solutions. Rather, even the final question (v. 31) confronts a reader with her or his own assumptions. The assumption of this reading was explained early on in this study. As the analysis of the ideas on rape in biblical scholarship and the exegesis demonstrated, readers are substantially implicated in the interpretation. Views regarding rape determine how readers evaluate the ensuing events, including the fraternal revenge.

Third, the interpretation makes a connection between the rape and the revenge. Often biblical scholars considered the revenge to be worse than the rape. Some disconnected the two; others minimized the rape and emphasized the revenge. In contrast, this feminist interpretation sees an inextricable tie between the rape and the revenge. I argue that the revenge is the original form of violence in the story. The understanding of rape as a severe problem in contemporary Western societies deepens a reader's sensibility about the grief of the brothers. Their concern for their sister leads to violent and bloody measure. They kill all the male Shechemites and capture the women and children. Thus, their reaction illustrates the societal dimensions of rape. Not only the rapist but the whole town participates in rape-prone behavior. Feminist scholarship highlights this understanding of rape. The brothers' revenge, however, also demonstrates their conflicting views about women. On the one hand they defend their sister. On the other hand they do not hesitate to capture other women as if these women were

---

[93] A contemporary controversy about marriage after rape emerges currently in several Latin American countries. See a report in the *New York Times* (March 12, 1997): A1, A12: "Justice in Peru: Victim Gets Rapist for a Husband."

their booty. The connection of the rape and the resulting revenge clarifies that no easy solutions are available to stop rapists and rape-prone behavior. In this regard Genesis 34 invites contemporary readers to address the prevalence of rape through the metaphoric language of a story.

Chapter 7

Conclusion

To this day, only about half of the rapists in New York City but more than 85 percent of murderers are convicted.[1] Rape continues to be perceived as an excusable crime. The sources examined in this book speak to this trend. Selected from two different time periods, nineteenth-century Germany and the contemporary period, interpretations of Genesis 34 did not express rejection and disapproval for the rape or the rapist. Instead they distracted the attention from the crime in different ways.

Certainly, this biblical narrative contains complicating factors. Only the first verses report the events of the rape. The quantitative larger part describes the aftermaths. Supposedly Shechem changes his mind and wants to marry Dinah; negotiations and revenge follow. Ending with a question by Dinah's brothers, this biblical story does not clearly advise how best to respond. Should one stand with the brothers or with Jacob? What about the killing of all male Shechemites? Does the marriage proposal redeem the rape? What is a reader to think about this story?

Raised by the open-ended nature of Genesis 34, these questions make an analysis of scholarly interpretations fascinating. Voluntarily or not, readers give clear answers. In order to make sense of the complex events they choose and take sides. The examination of commentaries and articles presents their choices and stances. The description shows that biblical scholarship connects to the pervasiveness of rape in contemporary societies. Of course, the study does not want nor can establish direct or causative links. Nevertheless, the analysis relates

---

[1] "Rape Resists the Inroads Of the City's War on Crime," *New York Times* (August 23, 1998), 31.

biblical scholarship to a much larger societal problem. This connection presents in itself an exciting and invigorating step for biblical research. The conclusion discusses five areas which characterize the relationship: biblical cultural studies, perspective, methodology, Genesis 34, and feminist scholarship on rape.

Biblical Cultural Studies

Biblical researchers maintain that the Bible and biblical scholarship shaped Western culture, and cultural studies offer the opportunity to prove it. This study participates in the endeavor. It also confirms that the establishment of links between the Bible and culture energizes biblical scholarship. By crossing established disciplinary boundaries, the academic study of the Bible explores its ties to the larger cultural discourse. This book analyzes the relation between one particular text, one subject matter, and two time periods: Genesis 34, rape, and nineteenth-century and contemporary biblical scholarship. Part of the larger feminist and academic effort to illuminate the numerous ways rape has been conceptualized within Western societies, this book represents an important aspect in the larger discourse. It shows how a particular section of biblical scholarship has contributed to contemporary views on rape. Since biblical scholarship and its concepts shaped the theological and societal views of ministers and teachers, such research has been highly influential. It is, therefore, painful to confront the views on rape in the interpretations of Genesis 34.

The book explores ideas on rape from the nineteenth century and the contemporary period. Assuming that time and place informed biblical research, the study compares views of commentaries with those of forensic textbooks from nineteenth-century Germany. The pairing shows that the commentaries and the forensic medical textbooks shared a common discourse. They did not consider rape a topic in its own right. Rape became an opportunity for male bonding against the woman and those who sided with her. Scholars claimed that love and libido resulted from rape. They also maintained that the age of the woman relativized the severity of rape. The emphasis on other issues, such as Orientalism or virginity, diverted the significance of the rape. The examination of biblical scholarship from nineteenth-century German profited from the juxtaposition. Links were established that otherwise would not appear. A partial "network of interests" between theological and scientific treatments of rape during nineteenth-century Germany became visible.

The examination of contemporary readings of Genesis 34 gives reason for concern. Biblical scholars marginalize the rape to focus on the male characters of the story. They do not discuss sexual violence or the relation between rape and hierarchical structures of society. The narrative turns into a love story and a story about Israelite tribal history. Labeled feminist, several interpretations neglect the rape in similar ways. Analyzed with a contemporary feminist perspective, the interpretations do not take into account the observations made by feminist research. In contrast to the perspective defined by feminist scholarship, contemporary interpretations—feminist or not—do not side with Dinah. Similar to nineteenth-century readings, they marginalize the rape.

An exegesis restores this imbalance. Using a literary method endebted to rhetorical criticism, the exegetical chapter reads Genesis 34 as Dinah's story. Five scenes divide the narrative. Scene One describes the rape (vv. 1-3), Scene Two reports the reaction (vv. 4-7), Scene Three presents the negotiations (vv. 8-24), Scene Four the killing (vv. 25-29), and Scene Five the conversation between Jacob and his two sons Simeon and Levi (vv. 30-31).

As a cultural study, this work includes only a small number of cultural resources. Other cultural artifacts exist that could further illustrate the connections between the discourse on rape in biblical scholarship and its settings. Therefore, the exploration here constitutes only a fragment of larger dynamics at work when readers interpret Genesis 34. Biblical cultural studies constitute an excellent forum in which such research can be done.

Perspective

The study employs a feminist perspective defined by feminist scholarship. Feminist research emphasizes rape and the situation of victim-survivors. Rape is regarded as sexual violence and understood within institutional and societal structures of hierarchy and discrimination. Feminists differentiate between various forms of rape and connect it to other oppressive conditions, so that it turns into a global issue. Defining rape accordingly, the present study does not claim objectivity or neutrality in the general sense of these two words. "One is always *somewhere*, and limited." Thus, an analysis from a particular and specific location promises "more adequate, sustained, objective, transforming accounts of the world."[2] Here a feminist perspective examines the views on rape in interpretations of Genesis 34.

Biblical scholarship shows concern into developing situated discourse in which an exegete discloses her or his perspective. Numerous publications indicate the demand for readings from different perspectives shaped by gender, race, ethnicity, or nationality.[3] Feminist standpoint theorists point out, however, that not all perspectives are equally valid. One has to identify criteria that allow to evaluate what view is preferred under the particular circumstances. According to Donna J. Haraway, generally "the standpoints of the subjugated . . . are preferred." These standpoints require a "critical examination" because they too are "not [an] 'innocent' position."[4] Hence, this study analyzes interpretations from a feminist, i.e., the raped woman's, view as theorized in feminist scholarship.

Biblical scholar Gary A. Philipps proposes a similar criterion for evaluating the perspective of an interpretation. He suggests to consider the ethical implications of one's work.[5] According to this criterion, interpreters have to reflect upon the ethics of their readings, so that ethical concerns become a central part of the interpretive process.[6] In the arena of biblical cultural studies, such a consideration promises challenging and stimulating discussions. The present work participates in the endeavor. Analyzing ideas on rape in interpretations of Genesis 34 and exegeting this narrative as "Dinah's story," the study recommends that future conversations on Genesis 34 take seriously the issue of rape from a feminist stance.

---

[2] See footnote 34 in Chapter One.

[3] See the increasing number of publications in biblical cultural studies as listed in footnotes 14-21 in chapter 1.

[4] See footnote 40 in chapter 1.

[5] He proposed this standard in his talk at the session "African-American Theology and Biblical Hermeneutics Group: Ideological Criticism Group" of the meeting of the *Society of Biblical Literature* in 1996.

[6] For other and earlier considerations of ethics as a part of the interpretive process see the works cited in footnote 27 in chapter 1.

Methodology

The study uses a variety of methods. The examination relies on intertextual reading strategies as explored by secular and religious-theological scholarship. Scholars use them to integrate different materials for analyzing the subject matters and for creating connections that provide new understandings. In the case of nineteenth-century interpretations and forensic medicine the approach leads to informative connections. Sometimes, however, the finding of comparable elements is not so easy. A careful study of the concepts as well as an extended immersion into the arguments is required to create relationships between the prevailing concepts.[7]

At the same time the interdisciplinary reading strategies expand possible conversations between various academic disciplines that have rarely interacted in the history of biblical scholarship. A stimulation of such an exchange is necessary in a time of complexity and uncertainty. Moreover, biblical scholars profited from interdisciplinary work in the past. For instance, archaeological discoveries, ancient Near Eastern literatures, and linguistics have shaped biblical research during the last centuries. Biblical scholars indicate now an interest in anthropology.[8] The consultation of interdisciplinary materials has thus been an integral part of biblical studies.

Besides these strategies, the exegetical chapter applies rhetorical criticism to exegete Genesis 34. As a literary method, rhetorical criticism investigates the final textual form and searches for literary features in the text, constituting the formal elements. Rhetorical criticism provides numerous literary components that strengthen the reading of Genesis 34 as a rape story. The exegesis demonstrates that the narrative can be read as an entity in itself that does not necessarily relate to the Jacob-cycle. In fact, limited to one chapter, Genesis 34 emerges as a dramatic discussion about the dilemma of negotiating two violent acts, the rape and the ensuing vengeful killing. According to the rhetorical analysis all other scenes follow from the rape, the central event

---

[7] For a recognition of this problem for cross-cultural studies see Victor H. Matthews and Don C. Benjamin, "Social Sciences and Biblical Studies," *Semeia:* Honor and Shame in the World of the Bible 18 (1996): 17-18.

[8] See the volume of *Semeia:* Honor and Shame in the World of the Bible 68 (1996).

of the narrative. Literary allusions to the rape (e.g. v. 13), the presence of Dinah throughout the narrative in many pronouns and references to her person, and the repetitive arrangements of the speeches
(e.g. vv. 9, 16, 21) attest to its centrality.

Feminist scholarship provides further insights for the interpretation. Often such research appears only in the background and serves
as a guideline to the events. The goal is here to integrate feminist
discourse into the exegesis. Therefore, short references tie feminist
scholarship to the specific passage at the end of each interpretive
section. For instance, the characterization of Shechem as a "sexual
gratification rapist" establishes a direct parallel. Other relations remain more subtle (e.g., vv. 4-7). As a result, the reading is not dominated but informed by feminist research.

Genesis 34

Interpreters read Dinah's story with manifold concepts of rape. The
analysis of the history of interpretation shows that not one single unequivocal topic emerges. Interpreters focus on, for example, the various male characters, tribal history, love, xenophobia, or source critical
issues. They do not stress the rape or Dinah. The exegetical chapter
presents such an emphasis. Grounded in rhetorical criticism, the reading suggests that the rape and Dinah are rhetorically central. Genesis
34 is a rape story and the literary features of the text support this
conclusion.

The question arises whether another rhetorical interpretation could
lead to a different emphasis from rape and Dinah. Theoretically, such
an alternative makes sense because the history of interpretation demonstrates that many different foci are applied to the text. At the same
time rhetorical critics maintain that rhetorical criticism uncovers the
literary features of a text. Thus the text itself sets limits to countless
alternatives.[9] It remains to be seen whether an alternative would sufficiently include the literary features and integrate them into a focus
that is not the rape or Dinah.

The exegesis also illuminates that the issue of shame and honor
does not play a significant role although scholars apply this anthropo-

---

[9] For this argument see Phyllis Trible, *Rhetorical Criticism: Context, Method,
and the Book of Jonah* (Minneapolis: Fortress Press, 1994), 231.

logical concept to the narrative.[10] The vocabulary of the text does not use the terminology that refers to shame and honor. Words such as בוש or כלם for shame and כבד for honor do not appear in Genesis 34. Anthropologist John K. Chance reponds critically to applying anthropological concepts to biblical texts. He remarks that the simple application of anthropological concepts, such as shame and honor, does not suffice.[11] Complex and disputed among anthropologists, these concepts have to be situated within the cultural, social, and political context of their society. Examined with other historical materials of that setting, anthropological categories might then explain certain customs in ancient Israel. However, the problems of establishing such a historical context are well-known. The authorship of biblical books and passages are usually unknown or multiple; the dating is often vague. Both problems pertain to Genesis 34 where neither the authorship nor the dating is clear. Hence, Chance maintains that "enthusiasm for ethnography must not be allowed to result in the neglect of historical evidence, vague and incomplete as it often is."[12] In other words, without a precise knowedge about the historical conditions that brought forth Genesis 34, anthropological concepts should be applied "very carefully" because "we may never know for sure"[13] the historical circumstances.

The dilemma of two acts of violence constitutes another issue that biblical scholars have faced. They recognize that the rape and the vengeful killing require evaluative statements. Most often, they consider the rape as less severe than the killing of the male town inhabitants. Thus, they reprimand the brothers for their brutal revenge and marginalize the rape. In contrast, the exegesis of this study integrates

---

[10] For an explanation of Genesis 34 under this category see Lyn M. Bechtel, "What if Dinah Is not Raped? (Genesis 34)," *Journal for the Study of the Old Testament* 62 (1994): 19-36. For general discussions within biblical scholarship see the essays in *Semeia* 68 (1996); Lyn M. Bechtel, "Shame as a Sanction of Social Control in Biblical Israel: Judicial, Political, and Social Shaming," *Journal for the Study of the Old Testament* 49 (February 1991): 47-76; Saul M. Olyan, "Honor, Shame, and Covenant Relations in Ancient Israel and Its Environment," *Journal of Biblical Literature* 115, no. 2 (1996): 201-218.

[11] John K. Chance, "The Anthropology of Honor and Shame: Culture, Values, and Practice," *Semeia* 68: Honor and Shame in the World of the Bible (1996): 140-141.

[12] Ibid., 142.

[13] Ibid., 142, 147.

both acts while it emphasizes the importance of the rape and hence Dinah. The interpretation acknowledges the ethical problems involved in the revenge. On the one hand, the brothers stay in a mindset that differentiates between "our" and "their" women; the brothers defend only Dinah. On the other hand, they do not confine their anger to the rapist. Interpreted in conjunction with feminist scholarship, the brothers seem to recognize the societal complicity that tolerates and supports rape-prone behavior. Further, the exegetical chapter maintains that the narrative depicts rape as the cause for the revenge. Although both elements shape the story, the rape is the reason for telling it. Genesis 34 is Dinah's story.

Feminist Scholarship on Rape

This study documents that interpretations of Genesis 34 marginalize, subordinate, ignore, or misrepresente the rape or Dinah in various ways. Feminist scholarship provides intellectual and scholarly resources for this task. With all the volumes of feminist research on rape it is astounding that most readings on Genesis 34 rarely consider this body of scholarship. Feminist debate, therefore, continues to remain outside the research done on that story.

Two reasons might account for the exclusion. One refers to the understanding of biblical scholarship as a historical discipline. As such, biblical researchers do not mean to entertain contemporary questions and problems. Rather, they seek to reconstruct ancient Israelite history.[14] As a result, they claim that rape did not play the role in ancient Israelite society as it does today. Chapters 3 and 5 demonstrate that many interpreters argue this way. Another approach, however, is possible. Genesis 34 may be read as a narrative and not as a historical account. The metaphoric language of this story may then contribute to contemporary reflection on the issue of rape. Such a reading profits from feminist work, as chapter 6 demonstrates.

The other reason pertains to a general reluctance to engage feminist research. Maybe the disapproval about positions taken in feminist studies leads researchers to ignore the enormous amount of feminist publications.[15] Hesitancy to open up biblical studies to a new field

---

[14] This understanding has been criticized see footnote 104 in chapter 5.

[15] Elaine Ginsberg and Sara Lennox, "Antifeminism in Scholarship and Publishing," in *Antifeminism in the Academy*, ed. VéVé Clark a.o. (New York: Routledge, 1996), 169-199.

might also account for the ease with which feminist theories have remained outside the scholarly research on Genesis 34. Interpreters can still ignore such discussions without wondering whether their work is complete. Instead, biblical scholars need to engage theories of feminist studies when they interpret stories of rape, even if they disagree with them. It seems that scholarly integrity requires that one takes advantage of scholarly works related to one's subject matter.

Ultimately, interpreters have to decide for whom they read Genesis 34. Whether they choose an interpretive stance because colleagues engage it or political and ethical reasons lead them to it, their interpretations are not read in an interest-free environment.[16] In the case of Genesis 34 interpretations advanced many rape plots that wronged Dinah. May the effort to uncover these plots contribute to changing a culture in which rapes occur daily.

---

[16] For an exploration of this dynamic see Stephen Fowl, "The Ethics of Interpretation or What's Left Over After the Elimination of Meaning," in *The Bible in Three Dimensions: Essays in Celebration of Forty Years of Biblical Studies in the University of Sheffield*, ed. David J. A. Clines a. o. (Sheffield: Sheffield Academic Press, 1990), 380-398.

Appendix

Law Codes on Rape of Nineteenth-Century Germany

Law Codes until 1870

From: Friedrich Wilhelm Bocker, *Lehrbuch der gerichtlichen Medicin: mit Berücksichtigung der gesammten deutschen und rheinischen Gesetzgebung als Leitfaden zu seinen Vorlesungen und zum Gebrauch für Aerzte und Juristen*, 2nd rev. and exp. ed. (Iserlohn, Badeker, 1857), 263-267.

§. 106. Die gesetzwidrige Geschlechtsbefriedigung.

A. Gesetzliche Bestimmungen.

a. Preussen.

§. 143. Die widernatürliche Unzucht, welche zwischen Personen männlichen Geschlechts oder von Menschen mit Thieren verübt wird, ist mit Gefängniss von sechs Monaten bis zu vier Jahren, so wie mit zeitiger Untersagung der Ausübung der bürgerlichen Ehrenrechte zu bestrafen.

§. 144. Mit Zuchthaus bis zu zwanzig Jahren wird bestraft: 1) wer an einer Person des einen oder des andern Geschlechtes mit Gewalt eine auf Befriedigung des Geschlechtstriebes gerichtete unzüchtige Handlung verübt, oder sie durch Drohungen mit gegenwärtiger Gefahr für Leib oder Leben zu Duldung einer solchen unzüchtigen Handlung zwingt; 2) wer eine, in einem willenlosen oder bewusstlosen Zustande befindliche Person zu einer auf Befriedigung des Geschlechtstriebes gerichteten unzüchtigen Handlung missbraucht; 3) wer mit Personen unter vierzehn Jahren unzüchtige Handlungen vornimmt, oder dieselben zur Verübung oder Duldung unzüchtiger Handlungen verleitet. — Ist der Tod der Person, gegen welche das Verbrechen geübt wird, dadurch verursacht worden, so tritt lebenslängliche Zuchthausstrafe ein.

b. Oesterreich.

§. 125. Wer eine Frauensperson durch gefährliche Drohung, wirklich ausgeübte Gewältthätigkeit oder durch arglistige Betäubung ihrer Sinne ausser Stand setzt, ihm Widerstand zu thun, und sie in diesem Zustande zu ausserehelichem Beischlafe missbraucht, begeht das Verbrechen der Nothzucht.

§. 126. Die Strafe der Nothzucht ist schwerer Kerker zwischen fünf und zehn Jahren. Hat die Gewaltthätigkeit einen wichtigen Nachtheil der Beleidigten an ihrer Gesundheit, oder gar am Leben zur Folge gehabt, so soll die Strafe auf eine Dauer zwischen zehn und zwanzig Jahren verlängert werden. Hat das Verbrechen den Tod der Beleidigten verursacht, so tritt lebenslanger Kerker ein.

§. 127. Der an einer Frauensperson, die sich ohne Zuthun des Thäters im Zustande der Wehr- oder Bewusstlosigkeit befindet, oder noch nicht das vierzehnte Lebensjahr erreicht hat, unternommene ausscheheliche Beischlaf, ist gleichfalls als Nothzucht anzusehen, und nach §. 126 zu bestrafen.

§. 128. Wer einen Knaben oder ein Mädchen unter vierzehn Jahren oder eine im Zustande der Wehr- oder Bewusstlosigkeit befindliche Person zur Befriedigung seiner Lüste auf eine andere als die im §. 127 bezeichnete Weise geschlechtlich missbraucht, begeht, wenn diese Handlung nicht das im §. 129 I. Lit. b. bezeichnete Verbrechen bildet, das Verbrechen der Schändung, und soll mit schwerem Kerker von einem bis fünf Jahren, bei sehr erschwerenden Umständen bis zu zehn, und wenn eine der im §. 126 erwähnten Folgen eintritt, bis zu zwanzig Jahren bestraft werden.

§. 129. Als Verbrechen werden auch nachstehende Arten von Unzucht bestraft:
I. Unzucht wider die Natur, das ist
    a. mit Thieren,
    b. mit Personen desselben Geschlechts.

c. Baiern. Oldenburg.

Vollendete Nothzucht (sobald die körperliche Vereinigung wirklich erfolgt ist) an einer Frauens- oder Mannsperson verübt, nach dem oben bei Oesterreich angegebenen Begriffe, trifft Arbeitshaus von vier bis acht Jahren, verbunden mit jährlicher einsamer Einsperrung in dem Zuchthause (Art. 186 und 187 Thl. I.). Wenn aber die Nothzucht an einem Menschen unter zwölf Jahren begangen worden ist, oder wenn die genothzüchtigte Person durch die verübte Gewalt, oder durch den Beischlaf selbst an ihrer Gesundheit irgend einen Nachtheil erlitten, so erfolgt acht- bis zehnjähriges Zuchthaus. (Art. 188 Thl. I.) Ist die genothzüchtigte Person an den Misshandlungen gestorben, so wird der Verbrecher am Leben bestraft (Art. 189 Thl. I.). Wer eine Person durch arglistige Betäubung ihrer Sinne ausser Stand setzt, seine Lüste abzuwehren, und dieselbe in diesem Zustande zur Befriedigung der Wollust missbraucht, hat ein- bis vierjähriges Arbeitshaus verwirkt. (Art. 190 Thl. I.) Wer eine wahnsinnige, blödsinnige, schlafende oder höchst betrunkene Person zur Befriedigung seiner Wollust missbraucht, verwirkt dreimonatliches bis zweijähriges Gefängniss. (Art. 377 Thl. I.) Der Beischlaf mit einem Mädchen unter zwölf Jahren ist von ihrer Seite als unfreiwillige Unzucht zu betrachten, und soll an dem Verführer mit sechsmonatlicher bis zweijährigem Gefängniss bestraft werden, sofern nicht die Handlung wegen verübter Gewalt oder Drohungen in das Verbrechen der Nothzucht übergegangen ist (Art. 378 Thl. I.).

d. Sachsen. Altenburg.

Nothzucht. Wer eine Frauensperson durch äussere Gewalt, welche nach den vorliegenden Umständen von ihr nicht abgewendet werden konnte, oder durch eine, mit gegenwärtiger, gleichfalls unabwendbarer Gefahr für Leben oder Gesundheit verbundene Drohung zur Duldung unehelichen Beischlafs nöthigt, wird mit sechs- bis zehnjähriger Zuchthausstrafe ersten Grades (Altenburg: mit sieben bis zwölfjähriger und, wenn die genothzüchtigte Person vorher in dem begründeten Rufe einer unzüchtigen und liederlichen Lebensart gestanden hat, mit ein- bis fünfjähriger Zuchthausstrafe belegt (Art. 157). Gleiche Strafe hat derjenige verwirkt, welcher unter Anwendung solcher Gewalt oder Drohung eine Frauens- oder Mannsperson zur naturwidrigen Befriedigung des Geschlechtstriebes missbraucht. (Art. 158). Hat bei einer von Einem oder Mehreren verübten Nothzucht die gemisshandelte Person einen bleibenden Nachtheil an ihrer Gesundheit erlitten, oder ist der Tod derselben durch die verübte Nothzucht verursacht worden, so ist die Zuchthausstrafe verhältnissmässig zu verlängern, und kann im letzten Falle bis zu zwanzig Jahren gesteigert werden. (Art. 159). Unzucht mit Personen im bewusstlosen Zustande. Wer eine Frauensperson, die in einem bewusstlosen Zustande sich befindet, zur Befriedigung der Wollust missbraucht, ist mit Zuchthaus (Sachsen zweiten Grades) von einem bis zu zwei Jahren zu belegen. Hat der Verbrecher den bewusstlosen Zustand absichtlich zu Erreichung dieses Zweckes herbeigeführt, so findet zwei- bis fünfjährige Zuchthausstrafe ersten Grades (Altenburg, drei- bis sechsjährige Zuchthausstrafe) statt. Unzucht mit Kindern unter vierzehn Jahren. Diejenigen, welche Kinder unter zwölf Jahren zum Beischlafe missbrauchen, oder zu Aufreizung oder Befriedigung des Geschlechtstriebes andere unzüchtige Handlungen mit ihnen vornehmen, trifft ein- bis dreijähriges Zuchthaus (Sachsen zweiten Grades.). Ist dadurch ein bleibender Nachtheil für die Gesundheit des Kindes entstanden, so tritt vier- bis achtjährige Zuchthausstrafe ersten Grades (Altenburg, fünf- bis zehnjährige Zuchthausstrafe) ein; hat die Misshandlung den Tod des Kindes zur Folge gehabt, so ist die Strafe auf zehn- bis fünfzehnjähriges Zuchthaus ersten Grades (Altenburg, auf zwölf- bis achtzehnjähriges Zuchthaus) zu erhöhen. — Wer mit einer Frauensperson über zwölf jedoch unter vierzehn Jahren alt Unzucht treibt, wird mit vier bis sechs Monaten Gefängniss belegt. Hat die gemissbrauchte Person dadurch einen bleibenden Nachtheil an ihrer Gesundheit erlitten, so tritt Arbeitshaus bis zu drei Jahren ein; ist dadurch der Tod der Gemissbrauchten verursacht worden, so kann die Strafe bis auf vier Jahr Zuchthaus (Sachsen zweiten Grades) gesteigert werden. (Art 161.) Die in den Artikeln 157, 158, 159 und 160 aufgeführten Verbrechen, sowie alle andere fleischliche (Altenburg: geschlechtliche) Verbrechen, sind für vollendet zu erachten, sobald die körperliche Vereinigung erfolgt ist. (Art. 162).

Von der widernatürlichen Befriedigung des Geschlechtstriebes handelt Art. 308.

e. Würtemberg.

Wer eine Frauensperson durch körperliche Gewalt, gefährliche Drohung oder arglistige Betäubung ihrer Sinne ausser Stand setzt, seinen Lüsten Widerstand zu leisten, und in solchem Zustande sie schändet, wird wegen Nothzucht bestraft: 1) mit lebenslänglichem Zuchthaus, wenn der Tod der genothzüchtigten Person durch die erlittene Misshandlung verursacht worden ist; 2) mit Zuchthaus nicht unter zehn Jahren, wenn die genothzüchtigte Person an ihrer Gesundheit einen bleibenden Nachtheil erlitten hat; 3) ausserdem mit vierjährigem Arbeitshaus bis fünfzehnjährigem Zuchthaus. — Gleiche Strafe, nach dem im vorigen Artikel festgesetzten Unterschiede, hat derjenige verwirkt, welcher eine Frauens- oder Mannsperson zur naturwidrigen Befriedigung des Geschlechtstriebes durch Anlegung von Gewalt, gefährliche Bedrohung oder arglistige Betäubung ihrer Sinne gemissbraucht hat. (Art. 296). Wer eine Person, die das vierzehnte Lebensjahr noch nicht zurückgelegt hat, zur Unzucht missbraucht, ist nach Verschiedenheit der im §. 295 genannten Fälle mit den auf die Nothzucht gesetzten Strafen zu belegen; sollte sich jedoch ergeben, dass eine zu solchem Zwecke missbrauchte Frauensperson schon mannbar gewesen ist, so kann im Falle der Nr. 3 des Art. 295 bis zum niedrigsten Masse des Arbeitshauses herabgestiegen werden. — Ist gegen die Person Gewalt (Art. 295.) gebraucht worden, so darf auf keine geringere, als die in Nr. 2 des erwähnten Artikels bestimmte Strafe erkannt werden. (Art. 297). Wer eine wahnsinnige, blödsinnige oder im Zustande der Betäubung befindliche Person zur Befriedigung der Wollust missbraucht, wird mit Kreisgefängniss bestraft. (Art. 299). Von der widernatürlichen Unzucht handelt Artikel 310.

f. Braunschweig. Detmold.

Nothzucht. Wer gegen eine Frauensperson Gewalt oder gefährliche Drohungen anwendet, oder sie in einen Zustand der Betäubung versetzt, um sie zur Duldung des unehelichen Beischlafs zu nöthigen, erleidet: 1) Kettenstrafe bis von zehn Jahren, wenn der Angriff lebensgefährlich war, oder wenn Mehrere die That gemeinschaftlich verübten, oder wenn die Angegriffene das fünfzehnte Jahr nicht überschritten hatte und in allen diesen Fällen ausserdem die verbrecherische Absicht erreicht ist; 2) Zuchthaus in andern Fällen jedoch nicht unter drei Jahren, wenn auch nur einer der im vorigen Absatze aufgeführten erschwerenden Umstände eintritt, oder die verbrecherische Absicht erreicht worden. (§. 172). Wer eine Frauens- oder Mannsperson durch Gewalt oder gefährliche Drohungen, oder, nachdem er sie in einen Zustand der Betäubung versetzt hat, zur naturwidrigen Befriedigung des Geschlechtstriebes missbraucht, soll einem Nothzüchtiger gleich bestraft werden (Art. 173). Schändung. Wer eine wahnsinnige, blödsinnige oder in einem bewusstlosen Zustande ohne sein Verschulden befindliche Person zur Befriedigung des Geschlechtstriebes missbraucht, verwirkt Zwangsarbeit nicht unter einem Jahre.

g. Hannover.

Nothzucht. Begriff wie oben bei Braunschweig §. 172, Art. 270. Der Nothzüchtiger ist mit geschärftem Zuchthaus nicht unter vier Jahren, oder Kettenstrafe bis zu fünfzehn Jahren zu belegen. — Ist jedoch I. die Nothzucht an einem noch nicht mannbaren Mädchen verübt, oder hat die genothzüchtigte Person durch die That an ihrer Gesundheit einen bedeutenden Nachtheil erlitten, so findet Kettenstrafe von acht bis zu zwanzig Jahren statt. II. Wenn der Tod der genothzüchtigten Person durch die Misshandlungen verursacht worden, so soll der Verbrecher, falls nicht seine That als vorsätzliche Tödtung sich darstellt, zu lebenslänglicher Kettenstrafe verurtheilt werden (Art. 271). Schändung. Wer eine Frauensperson, die sich in einem die Willensfreiheit aufhebenden Zustande, eines Gemüthsgebrechens, einer Ohnmacht, Betäubung oder sonstigen Bewusstlosigkeit befindet, zum Beischlafe missbraucht, der ist der Schändung schuldig, und soll mit Zuchthaus, und bei besonders mildernden Umständen, mit Arbeitshaus bestraft werden. —

h. Hessen.

Nothzucht. Begriff wie oben bei Würtemberg im Art. 295 (Art. 329). Strafe 1) wenn die genothzüchtigte Person in Folge der erlittenen Misshandlung gestorben ist, Zuchthaus auf Lebenszeit; 2) wenn die genothzüchtigte Person durch die That an ihrer Gesundheit bedeutenden Nachtheil erlitten hat, Zuchthaus von acht bis sechszehn Jahren; 3) in allen andern Fällen Zuchthaus bis zu zehn Jahren (Art. 330). Verführung zur Unzucht. Wer eine Frauensperson, welche das vierzehnte Lebensjahr noch nicht zurückgelegt hat, zur Unzucht verführt und missbraucht, ist, nach Verschiedenheit der im Art. 330 genannten Fälle mit den auf die Nothzucht gesetzten Strafen zu belegen. — Die im vorigen Artikel angedrohten Strafen treffen auch eine Person, welche einen noch nicht 14 Jahre alten Knaben zur Unzucht verführt und dieselbe mit ihm verübt (Art. 332). Correctionshaus bis zu drei, oder Zuchthaus bis zu vier Jahren trifft Denjenigen, welcher eine wahnsinnige, blödsinnige oder in dem Zustande der Betäubung, sowie in einem sonst willens- oder bewusstlosen Zustande befindliche Person schändet (Art. 334). In allen Fällen, in welchen die Unzucht durch Beischlaf verübt wird, ist das Verbrechen für vollendet zu achten, wenn körperliche Vereinigung erfolgt ist (Art. 342). Art. 338 handelt von widernatürlicher Unzucht.

i. Baden.

Nothzucht. Wer eine Frauensperson durch thätliche Gewalt, oder durch angewendete, mit der Gefahr unverzüglicher Verwirklichung verbundene Drohungen mit Tödtung oder schweren körperlichen Misshandlungen, gerichtet gegen sie selbst, oder gegen eine der im §. 81 bezeichneten Personen, zum unehelichen Beischlaf nöthig t, verwirkt folgende Strafen: I. Todesstrafe, wenn die Misshandlung den Tod der Genötbigten zur Folge hatte, insofern dem Thäter dieser Erfolg seiner Handlung zum bestimmten oder unbestimmten Vorsatz zuzurechnen ist; II. Lebenslängliches oder zeitliches Zuchthaus nicht unter zwölf Jahren: 1) wenn die Misshandlung, welche den, dem Thäter nicht zum Vorsatz zuzurechnenden, Tod der Genöthigten zur Folge hatte, von der Art war, dass der Tod von ihm als deren wahrscheinliche Folge vorher gesehen werden konnte; oder 2) wenn die Genöthigte an ihrem Körper oder ihrer Gesundheit eine, dem Thäter zum bestimmten oder unbestimmten Vorsatz zuzurechnende, schwere, bleibende Verletzung (Arbeitsunfähigkeit, Geisteszerrüttung, Beraubung eines Sinnes, einer Hand, eines Fusses, der Sprache oder Zeugungsfähigkeit) erlitten hat, oder die eingetretene Verletzung dieser Art von ihm als eine wahrscheinliche Folge der Misshandlung vorhergesehen werden konnte; III. Zuchthaus nicht unter sechs bis zu fünfzehn Jahren, wenn die Misshandlung, welche den, dem Thäter blos zur Fahrlässigkeit zuzurechnenden Tod der Genöthigten, oder eine ihm bloss zur Fahrlässigkeit zuzurechnende Verletzung der unter II. angegebenen Art zur Folge katte, von der Beschaffenheit war, dass der Tod oder die eingetretene Verletzung von ihm als deren wahrscheinliche Folge betrachtet werden konnte; IV. Zuchthaus bis zu zwölf Jahren, wenn die Genothzüchtigte an ihrem Körper oder ihrer Gesundheit eine dem Thäter zum Vorsatze oder zur Fahrlässigkeit zuzurechnende Verletzung, welche einen Theil des Körpers verstümmelt, auffallend verunstaltet, des Gebrauchs eines der Glieder oder Sinnenwerkzeuge beraubt oder zu den Berufsarbeiten bleibend unfähig macht, erlitten hat; V. in andern Fällen, wenn die Genöthigte in Ansehung der Geschlechtsehre von unbescholtenem Rufe ist, Zuchthaus bis zu acht Jahren, ausserdem Arbeitshaus nicht unter einem Jahre (§. 335). Die Strafen der Nothzucht treten ebenfalls ein: 1) gegen Denjenigen, der den Beischlaf mit einer Frauensperson vollzieht, welche er zu diesem Ende arglistiger Weise durch Mittel, die er ohne ihr Wissen beibrachte, oder durch Mittel, die er zwar mit ihrem Wissen beibrachte, aber deren Wirkung ihr unbekannt war, ausser Stand gesetzt hat, seinen Lüsten zu widerstehen; 2) gegen Denjenigen, der den Beischlaf mit einem Mädchen vollzieht, welches noch das 14. Lebensjahr nicht zurück gelegt hat, und noch nicht mannbar ist. (§. 336). Wer ohne Anwendung von thätlicher Gewalt, oder von Drohungen der im §. 335 bezeichneten Art, wissentlich eine wahnsinnige oder eine blödsinnige, oder eine sonst in einem willen- oder bewusslosen Zustande befindliche Frauensperson, die er nicht in diesen Zustand versetzt hat, zum Beischlafe missbraucht, wird mit Kreisgefängniss oder Arbeitshaus bestraft (§. 337).

k. Weimar-Eisenach. Meiningen. Coburg. Gotha. Anhalt-Dessau und Köthen. Rudolstadt. Sondershausen. Reuss.

Wer eine Frauensperson durch Anwendung von Gewalt, welche den Umständen nach nicht abgewendet werden konnte, oder durch Drohungen mit gegenwärtiger Gefahr für Leben oder Gesundheit, zur Duldung ausserehelichen Beischlafs nöthigt, verwirkt drei bis zehn Jahre Zuchthaus. Hat die gemissbrauchte Person durch die gegen sie angewandte Gewalt einen bleibenden Nachtheil an ihrer Gesundheit erlitten, oder ist ihr Tod durch die Nothzucht verursacht worden, so kann die Strafe bis zu zwanzigjähriger Zuchthausstrafe gesteigert werden. (Art. 292). Unzucht. Wer eine wahnsinnige, blödsinnige oder im bewusstlosen Zustande befindliche Frauensperson zum ausserehelichen Beischlaf gebraucht, hat Arbeitshaus oder Zuchthaus bis zu zwei Jahren verwirkt. — Hat er den bewusstlosen Zustand zum Behuf dieses Verbrechens selbst herbeigeführt, so findet zwei- bis fünfjährige Zuchthausstrafe statt. — Ist durch das Verbrechen ein bleibender Nachtheil für die Gesundheit oder der Tod der gemissbrauchten Person veranlasst worden, so trifft den Schuldigen sechs- bis zehnjähriges Zuchthaus. (Art. 296). Wer noch nicht mannbare Kinder unter 14 Jahren zum Beischlafe missbraucht, hat ein- bis dreijähriges, wenn aber ein bleibender Nachtheil für die Gesundheit des Kindes entstanden ist, vier- bis achtjähriges, und wenn seine That den Tod des Kindes zur Folge hatte, zehn- bis fünfzehnjähriges Zuchthaus verwirkt. (Art. 197). Wenn Jemand eine mannbare Person unter 14 Jahren, oder unter Anwendung von Betrug oder List eine andere unbescholtene Person zum Beischlaf mit sich verleitet, so tritt gegen den Verführer einmonatliche bis einjährige Gefängnissstrafe ein.

The Unified German Law Code of 1871

From: Eduard von Hofmann, *Lehrbuch der gerichtlichen Medicin: Mit besonderer Berücksichtigung der österreichischen und deutschen Gesetzgebung*, 5th rev. and exp. ed. (Vienna: Urban & Schwarzenberg, 1891), 99-100.

Deutsches Strafgesetz:

§. 173 Der Beischlaf zwischen Verwandten in auf- und absteigender Linie wird an den ersteren mit Zuchthaus bis zu 5 Jahren, an den letzteren mit Gefängniss bis zu 2 Jahren bestraft.

Der Beischlaf zwischen Verschwägerten auf- und absteigender Linie, sowie zwischen Geschwistern wird mit Gefängniss bis zu 2 Jahren bestraft.

§. 174. Mit Zuchthaus bis zu 5 Jahren werden bestraft:
1. Vormünder u. s. f.
2. Beamte u. s. f.
3. Beamte, Aerzte oder andere Medicinalpersonen, welche in Gefängnissen oder in öffentlichen, zur Pflege von Kranken, Armen oder anderen Hilfslosen bestimmten Anstalten beschäftigt oder angestellt sind, wenn sie mit den in das Gefängniss oder in die Anstalt aufgenommenen Personen unzüchtige Handlungen vornehmen.

Sind mildernde Umstände vorhanden, so tritt Gefängnissstrafe nicht unter 6 Monaten ein.

§. 175. Die widernatürliche Unzucht, welche zwischen Personen männlichen Geschlechtes oder von Menschen mit Thieren begangen wird, ist mit Gefängniss zu bestrafen; auch kann auf Verlust der bürgerlichen Ehrenrechte erkannt werden.

§. 176. Mit Zuchthaus bis zu 10 Jahren wird bestraft, wer
1. mit Gewalt unzüchtige Handlungen an einer Frauensperson vornimmt oder dieselbe durch Drohung mit gegenwärtiger Gefahr für Leib oder Leben zur Duldung unzüchtiger Handlungen nöthigt,
2. eine in einem willenlosen oder bewusstlosen Zustande befindliche oder geisteskranke Frauensperson zum ausserehelichen Beischlafe missbraucht, oder
3. mit Personen unter 14 Jahren unzüchtige Handlungen vornimmt, oder dieselben zur Verübung oder Duldung unzüchtiger Handlungen verleitet.

Sind mildernde Umstände vorhanden, so tritt Gefängnissstrafe nicht unter 6 Monaten ein.

Bibliography

Biblical Scholarship

Commentaries on Genesis of Nineteenth-Century Germany

Bachmann, Johannes, ed. *Praeparation und Commentar zur Genesis.* Berlin: Mayer & Müller, 1890-1893.

Baumgarten, Michael. *Theologischer Commentar zum Pentateuch.* Kiel: Universitäts-Buchhandlung, 1843.

Bohlen, P. von. *Die Genesis historisch-kritisch erläutert.* Königsberg: Gebrüder Bornträger, 1835

Bunsen, Christian Karl Josias Freiherr von. *Die Bibel oder die Schriften des Alten und Neuen Bundes nach dem überlieferten Grundtexten übersetzt und für die Gemeinde erklärt: Vollständiges Bibelwerk für die Gemeinde, in 3 Abtheilungen.* Erste Abtheilung: Die Bibel: Uebersetzung und Erklärung: Erster Theil: Das Gesetz. Leipzig: F. A. Brockhaus, 1858-1870.

Delitzsch, Franz Julius. *Die Genesis.* Leipzig: Dörffling & Franke, 1852.

————. *Die Genesis.* 2. Auflage. Leipzig: Dörffling & Franke, 1853.

————. *Neuer Commentar über die Genesis.* 5. verbesserte Auflage. Leipzig: Dörffling und Franke, 1887.

————. *A New Commentary on Genesis.* Translated by Sophia Taylor. 2 vols. Edinburgh: T. & T. Clark, 1889.

Dillmann, August. *Die Genesis.* Für die 3. Auflage nach Dr. August Knobel. Kurzgefasstes exegetisches Handbuch zum Alten Testament. Eilfte Lieferung. 3. verbesserte Auflage. Leipzig: S. Hirzel, 1875.

————. *Die Genesis.* 4. Auflage. Leipzig: S. Hirzel, 1882.

————. *Die Genesis.* Kurzgefasstes exegetisches Handbuch zum Alten Testament. 6. verbesserte Auflage. Leipzig: S. Hirzel, 1892.

Gunkel, Hermann. *Genesis*. Reihe Göttinger Handkommentar zum Alten Testament. 1. verbesserte Auflage. Göttingen: Vandenhoeck & Rupprecht, 1901.

Hoberg, Gottfried. *Die Genesis nach dem Literalsinn erklärt*. Freiburg im Breisgau: Herder, 1899.

Holzinger, Heinrich. *Genesis*. Kurzer Hand-Commentar zum Alten Testament. Freiburg/Leipzig/Tübingen: J.C.B. Mohr, 1898.

Kautzsch, Emil, and Albert Socin. *Die Genesis mit Äusserer Unterscheidung der Quellenschriften*. 2. verbesserte Auflage. Freiburg: J.C.B. Mohr, 1891.

Keil, Carl Friedrich. *Genesis und Exodus*. Biblischer Commentar über das alte Testament, ed. C. F. Keil and F. Delitzsch. Vol. 1. Leipzig: Dörffling & Franke, 1861.

———, and F. Delitzsch. *Biblical Commentary on the Old Testament*. Vol. 1: *The Pentateuch*. Translated by James Martin. Grand Rapids, MI: Eerdmans, 1949.

———, and Franz Delitzsch, eds. *The Pentateuch*. Biblical Commentary on the Old Testament. Vol. 1. Translated by James Martin. Grand Rapids, MI: Eerdmans, 1949.

Knobel, August. *Die Genesis*. Kurzgefasstes exegetisches Handbuch zum Alten Testament. Eilfte Lieferung. Leipzig: Weidmannsche Buchhandlung, 1852.

Kurtz, Johann Heinrich. *Die Einheit der Genesis: Ein Beitrag zur Kritik und Exegese der Genesis*. Berlin: Verlag von Justus Albert Wohlgemuth, 1846.

Lange, Johann Peter. *Die Genesis*. Theologisches-homiletisches Bibelwerk: Altes Testament. Bielefeld: Velhagen und Klasing, 1864.

———. *Genesis or the First Book of Moses together with a General Theological and Homiletical Introduction to the Old Testament*. Translated with additions by Taylor Lewis and A. Gosman. 5th rev. ed. New York: Charles Scribner, 1884.

Naumann, O. *Das Erste Buch der Bibel nach seiner inneren Einheit und Echtheit*. Gütersloh: C. Bertelsmann, 1890.

Schröder, Friedrich Wilhelm Julius. *Das erste Buch Mose*. Das Alte Testament nach Dr. Martin Luther: Mit Einleitungen, berichtigter Uebersetzung und erklärenden Anmerkungen: Für Freunde des göttlichen Wortes, mit bes. Rücksicht auf Lehrer in Kirchen und Schulen. Berlin: Justus Albert Wohlgemuth, 1846.

Strack, Hermann Leberecht. *Die Bücher Genesis, Exodus, Leviticus und Numeri*. Kurzgefasster Kommentar zu den heiligen Schriften

Alten und Neuen Testamentes sowie zu den Apokryphen: A. AT. 1. Abt. Hgs. H. Strack & Otto Zöckler. Munich: C. H. Beck, 1894.

Thiersch, Heinrich W. J. *Die Genesis nach ihrer moralischen und prophetischen Bedeutung*. Basel: Felix Schneider, 1870.

Tuch, Friedrich Johann Christian Friedrich. *Commentar über die Genesis*. 2. Auflage besorgt von A. Arnold, nebst einem Nachwort von A. Merz. Halle: Buchhandlung des Waisenhauses, 1871.

Vater, Johann Severin. *Commentar über den Pentateuch, mit Einleitung zu den einzelnen Abschnitten, der Eingeschalteten Uebersetzung von Dr. Alexander Geddes's Merkwürdigeren Critischen und exegetischen Anmerkungen und einer Abhandlung über Moses und die Verfasser des Pentateuchs.* 3 Vols. Halle: Waisenhaus Buchhandlung, 1802-1805.

Twentieth-Century Commentaries

Anderson, A. A. *The Book of Psalms*. New Century Bible. Vol. I. London: Marshall, Morgan & Scott, 1972.

Brueggemann, Walter. *Genesis: A Bible Commentary for Teaching and Preaching*. Atlanta: Knox Press, 1982.

Cassuto, U. *A Commentary on the Book of Genesis*. Translated by I. Abrahams. Part I: *From Adam to Noah Gen 1-6.8*. Jerusalem: Magnes Press, Hebrew University, 1978.

———. *Genesis: A Practical Commentary*. Translated by D. E. Green. Grand Rapids, MI: Eerdmans, 1987.

Clifford, Richard J., and Roland E. Murphy. "Genesis." Chap. in *The New Jerome Biblical Commentary*, ed. Raymond E. Brown, Joseph A. Fitzmyer, and Roland E. Murphy, 8-43. Englewood Cliffs, NJ: Prentice-Hall, 1990.

Coats, George W. *Genesis with an Introduction to Narrative Literature*. The Forms of the Old Testament Literature Series. Edited by Rolf Knierim and Gene M. Tucker. Vol. 1. Grand Rapids, MI: Eerdmans, 1983.

Davidson, Robert. *Genesis 12-50*. Cambridge Bible Commentary. Cambridge, UK: Cambridge University Press, 1979.

Hamilton, Victor P. *The Book of Genesis*. The New International Commentary on the Old Testament. Grand Rapids, MI: Eerdmans, 1995.

Jacob, Benno. *Das Erste Buch der Tora*. Berlin: Schocken, 1934.

Janzen, Gerald J. *Abraham and All the Families of the Earth: A Commentary on the Book of Genesis 12-50*. International Theological Commentary. Grand Rapids, MI: Eerdmans; Edinburgh: Handsel, 1993.

Leibowitz, Nehama. *Studies in Bereshit (Genesis): In the Context of Ancient and Modern Jewish Bible Commentary.* Translated and adapted by A. Newman. 2d rev. ed. Jerusalem: Jewish Agency at Haomanim, 1974.

Maher, Michael. *Genesis.* Wilmington, DE: Glazier, 1982.

Olyan, Saul M. "Honor, Shame, and Covenant Relations in Ancient Israel and Its Environment." *Journal of Biblical Literature* 115, no. 2 (1996): 201-18.

Rad, Gerhard von. *Genesis: A Commentary.* The Old Testament Library. Translated by John H. Marks. 3rd rev. ed. Philadelphia: Westminster Press, 1972.

Rudolph, Wilhelm. *Hosea.* Kommentar zum Alten Testament Series. Vol. 13. Gütersloh: Gütersloher Verlagshaus, 1966.

Sarna, Nahum M. *Genesis: The Traditional Hebrew Text with New JPS Translation.* JPS Torah Commentary Series. Philadelphia: Jewish Publication Society of America, 1989.

———. *Exodus.* The JPS Torah Commentary. Philadelphia: Jewish Publication Society, 1991.

Scharbert, Josef. *Genesis 12-50.* Würzburg: Echter Verlag, 1986.

Simpson, Cuthbert A., and Walter Russell Bowie. "Genesis." Chap. in *The Interpreter's Bible,* ed. George Buttrick. Vol. 1. Nashville: Abingdon Press, 1952, 26th Printing 1980.

Talbot, Gordon. *A Study of the Book of Genesis: An Introductory Commentary on All Fifty Chapters of Genesis.* Harrisburg, PA: Christian Publications, 1981.

Vawter, Bruce. *On Genesis: A New Reading.* Garden City, NY: Doubleday, 1977.

Weinfeld, Moshe. *The Book of Genesis.* Encyclopedia of the World of the Tanakh. Rabibim, 1982.

Wenham, Gordon J. *Genesis.* Word Biblical Commentary. Vol. 2. Waco, TX: Word Books, 1994.

Westermann, Claus. *Genesis 12-36: A Commentary.* Translated by J. J. Scullion. Minneapolis: Augsburg, 1985.

———. *Genesis 12-26: A Commentary.* Translated by J. J. Scullion. Minneapolis: Augsburg Press, 1985.

———. "נפש naefaes." In *Theologisches Handwörterbuch zum Alten Testament,* ed. Ernst Jenni and Claus Westermann, 71-96. Vol. 2. München: Kaiser, 1976.

Wolff, Hans Walter. *Micha: A Commentary.* Translated by Gary Stansell. Minneapolis: Augsburg Press, 1990.

Woods, Clyde M. *The Living Way Commentary on the Old Testament.* Vol. 1: *Genesis-Exodus.* Shreveport, LA: Lambert, 1972.

Articles, Essays, and Books of Biblical Scholarship

Aichele, George and Gary A. Philips, "Introduction, Exegesis, Eisegesis, Intergesis," *Semeia*: Intertextuality and the Bible 69/70 (1995): 7-18.

Alter, Robert. *The Art of Biblical Narrative.* New York: Basic Books, 1981.

———. *Genesis.* New York: W.W. Norton, 1996.

Amit, Jairah. "A Hidden Polemic in the Story of the Rape of Dinah (Hebrew)." In *Proceedings of the Eleventh World Congress of Jewish Studies.* Division A: *The Bible and Its World,* ed. David Assaf, 1-8. Jerusalem: Magnes Press, 1994.

———. "Hidden Polemic in the Conquest of Dan: Judges 17-18." *Vetus Testamentum* 60 (1990): 4-20.

André, G. "טמא tame.'" In *Theologisches Wörterbuch zum Alten Testament,* ed. Heinz-Josef Fabry and Helmer Ringgren, 352-66.Vol. 3. Stuttgart: Kohlhammer, 1982.

Antonelli, Judith S. *In the Image of God: A Feminist Commentary on the Torah.* Northvale, NJ: Jason Aronson, 1996.

Ararat, N. "Reading According to the 'Seder' in Biblical Narrative: To Balance the Reading of the Dinah Episode." *Hasifrut* 27 (1978): 15-34.

Armstrong, Karen. *In the Beginning: A New Interpretation of Genesis.* New York: Knopf, 1996.

Aschkenasy, Nehama. *Eve's Journey: Feminine Images in Hebraic Literary Tradition.* Philadelphia: University of Pennsylvania Press, 1986.

Bach, Alice. *Women, Seduction, and Betrayal in Biblical Narrative.* New York: Cambridge University Press, 1997.

Bailey, Clinton. "How Desert Culture Helps Us Understand the Bible: Bedouin Law Explains Reaction to Rape of Dinah." *Bible Review* 7, no. 4 (June 1991): 14-21, 38.

Bailey, D. S. *Homosexuality and the Western Christian Tradition.* London/New York: Longmans/Green, 1955.

Bar-Efrat, Shimon. "Time and Space." Chap. in *Narrative Art in the Bible*, Bible and Literature Series 17. Sheffield, UK: Sheffield Academic Press, 1989.

Bechtel, Lyn M. "What if Dinah Is not Raped? (Genesis 34)." *Journal for the Study of the Old Testament* 62 (1994): 19-36.

————. "Shame as a Sanction of Social Control in Biblical Israel: Judicial, Political, and Social Shaming." *Journal for the Study of the Old Testament* 49 (February 1991): 47-76.

Bechtoldt, Hans-Joachim. *Die jüdische Bibelkritik im 19. Jahrhundert*. Stuttgart: Kohlhammer, 1995.

Berquist, Jon L. *Reclaiming Her Story: The Witness of Women in the Old Testament*. St. Louis: Chalice Press, 1992.

Beuken, Wim, and Sean Freyne, eds. *The Bible as Cultural Heritage*. Concilium 1. Maryknoll, NY: Orbis, 1995.

Bible and Culture Collective. *The Postmodern Bible*. New Haven, CT: Yale University Press, 1995.

Bird, Phyllis. "'To Play the Harlot': An Inquiry into an Old Testament Metaphor." In *Gender and Difference in Ancient Israel*, ed. Peggy L. Day, 75-94. Minneapolis: Fortress, 1989.

————. "The Harlot as Heroine: Narrative Art and Social Presupposition in Three Old Testament Texts." *Semeia* 46 (1989): 119-39.

Blount, Brian K. *Cultural Interpretation: Reorienting New Testament Criticism*. Minneapolis: Fortress, 1995.

Blum, Erhard. *Die Komposition der Vätergeschichte*. Wissenschaftliche Monographien zum Alten und Neuen Testament. Vol. 57. Neukirchen-Vluyn: Neukirchener Verlag, 1984.

Botterweck, G. J. "חפץ ḥāpēṣ." In *Theologisches Wörterbuch zum Alten Testament*, ed. Ernst Jenni and Claus Westermann, 100-16.Vol. 3. Stuttgart: Kohlhammer, 1982.

Brisman, Leslie. *The Voice of Jacob: On the Composition of Genesis*. Bloomington: Indiana University Press, 1990.

Brown, Francis, S. R. Driver, and Charles A. Briggs, eds. *Hebrew and English Lexicon of the Old Testament, Based on the Lexicon of William Gesenius*. Oxford, UK: Oxford University Press, 1951.

Brueggemann, Walter. "Life and Death in Tenth Century Israel." *Journal of the American Academy of Religion* 40 (1972): 96-109.

Carmichael, C. M. *Women, Law, and the Genesis Tradition*. Edinburgh: Edinburgh University Press, 1979.

Chance, John K. "The Anthropology of Honor and Shame: Culture, Values, and Practice:" *Semeia: Honor and Shame in the World of the Bible* 68 (1996): 139-51.

Darr, Katheryn Pfisterer. *Far More Precious Than Jewels: Perspectives on Biblical Women.* Louisville, KY: Westminster/Knox Press, 1991.

Davis, John James. *Paradise to Prison: Studies in Genesis.* Grand Rapids, MI: Baker Book House, 1975.

Davies, Philip R. *In Search of 'Ancient Israel.'* Sheffield, UK: JSOT Press, 1992.

Diebner, Jörg Bernd. "Gen 34 und Dinas Rolle bei der Definition 'Israels.'" *Dielheimer Blätter zum Alten Testament* 19 (July 1984): 59-75.

Douglas, Mary. *In the Wilderness: The Doctrine of Defilement in the Book of Numbers.* Sheffield, UK: JSOT Press, 1993.

Dus, Jan. *Israelitische Vorfahren—Vasallen palästinischer Stadtstaaten? Revisionsbedürftigkeit der Landnahmehypothese von Albrecht Alt.* European University Studies 23. Vol. 404. Frankfurt: Lang, 1991.

Ehrlich, Arnold B. *Randglossen zur Hebräischen Bibel: Textkritisches, Sprachliches und Sachliches.* Vol. 5. Leipzig: Hinrich, 1912.

Erlandsson, E. "זנה zanah." In *Theologisches Wörterbuch zum Alten Testament,* ed. Heinz-Josef Fabry and Helmer Ringgren, 612-19. Vol. 2. Stuttgart: Kohlhammer, 1977.

Exum, J. Cheryl. "Feminist Criticism: Whose Interests Are Being Served?" In *Judges and Method: New Approaches in Biblical Studies,* ed. Gale A. Yee, 65-90. Minneapolis: Fortress, 1995.

————. *Plotted, Shot, and Painted: Cultural Representations of Biblical Women.* Sheffield: Sheffield Academic Press, 1996.

————. *Fragmented Women: Feminist (Sub)Versions of Biblical Narratives.* Valley Forge, PA: Trinity Press International, 1993.

Felder, Cain Hope, ed. *Stony the Road We Trod: African American Biblical Interpretation.* Minneapolis: Fortress, 1991.

Fewell, Danna Nolan, ed. *Reading between Texts: Intertextuality and the Hebrew Bible.* Louisville, KY: Westminster/Knox, 1992.

————, and David M. Gunn. "Tipping the Balance: Sternberg's Reader and the Rape of Dinah." *Journal of Biblical Literature* 110 (Summer 1991): 193-211.

Fields, Harvey J. *A Torah Commentary For Our Times*. Vol. 1: *Genesis*. New York: UAHC Press, 1990.

Fischer, Georg. "Die Redewendung דבר על לב im AT—Ein Beitrag zum Verständnis von Jes 40,2." *Biblica* 65 (1984): 244-50.

Fischer, Irmtraud. *Die Erzeltern Israels: Feministisch-theologische Studien zu Genesis 12-36*. Beihefte zur Zeitschrift für die alttestamentliche Wissenschaft, Bd. 222. Berlin: Walter de Gruyter, 1994.

Fishbane, Michael. "Composition and Structure in the Jacob Cycle (Gen. 25:19-35:22)." *Journal of Jewish Studies* 26 (1975): 15-38.

Fokkelman, J. P. *Narrative Art and Poetry in the Books of Samuel*. Vol. 1. Assen: Netherlands: Van Gorcum, 1981.

Fowl, Stephen. "The Ethics of Interpretation or What's Left Over After the Elimination of Meaning." In *The Bible in Three Dimensions: Essays in Celebration of Forty Years of Biblical Studies in the University of Sheffield*, eds. David J. A. Clines, Stephen E. Fowl, Stanley E. Porter, 379-98. Sheffield: Sheffield Academic Press, 1990.Fox, Everett. *In the Beginning: A New English Rendition of the Book of Genesis*. New York: Schocken, 1983.

Fox, Everett. *In the Beginning: A New English Rendition of the Book of Genesis*. New York: Schocken, 1983.

Freedman, D. N. "Dinah and Shechem: Tamar and Amnon." *Austin Seminary Bulletin: Faculty Edition* 105 (1990): 51-63.

Fretheim, Terence E. "The Book of Genesis: Introduction, Commentary, and Reflections." In *The New Interpreter's Bible*, ed. Leander E. Keck, 574-81. Vol. 1. Nashville, TN: Abingdon Press, 1994.

Friebe-Baron, Christine. *Ferne Schwestern, ihr seid mir nah: Begegnungen mit Frauen aus biblischer Zeit*. Stuttgart: Kreuz Verlag, 1988.

Frymer-Kensky, Tikva. "Law and Philosophy: The Case of Sex in the Bible." *Semeia* 45 (1989): 89-102.

———. "The Strange Case of the Suspected Sotah (Num. 5.11-31)." *Vetus Testamentum* 34/1 (1984): 11-26.

Fuchs, Esther. "Structure and Patriarchal Functions in the Biblical Betrothal Type-Scene: Some Preliminary Notes." *Journal of Feminist Studies in Religion* 3, no. 1 (Spring 1987): 7-13.

Fuhs, H. F. "נער na'ar." In *Theologisches Wörterbuch zum Alten Testament*, ed. Heinz-Josef Fabry and Helmer Ringgren, 507-18. Vol. 5. Stuttgart: Kohlhammer, 1986.

Geller, Stephen A. "The Sack of Shechem: The Use of Typology in Biblical Covenant." *Prooftexts* 10 (January 1990): 1-15.

Gerleman, G. "חפץ ḥpṣ." In *Theologisches Handwörterbuch zum Alten Testament*, ed. Ernst Jenni and Claus Westermann, 623-626. Vol. 1. München: Kaiser, 1971.

Gerstenberger, Erhard S. "ענה II 'anah." In *Theologisches Wörterbuch zum Alten Testament*, ed. Heinz-Josef Fabry and Helmer Ringgren, 247-70. Vol. 6. Stuttgart: Kohlhammer, 1989.

Gesenius, Wilhelm. *Hebräisches und Aramäisches Handwörterbuch über das Alte Testament*. Berlin: Springer, 1962.

Goodfriend, Elaine Adler. "Prostitution, Old Testament." In *The Anchor Bible Dictionary*. Vol. 5. New York: Doubleday, 1992.

Graetz, Naomi. "Dinah the Daughter." In *A Feminist Companion to Genesis*, ed. Athalia Brenner, 306-17. Sheffield, UK: JSOT, 1993.

Greenstein, Eduard L. *Essays on Biblical Method and Translation*. Brown Judaism Studies 92. Atlanta: Scholars Press, 1989.

Gruber, Mayer Irwin. *Aspects of Nonverbal Communication in the Ancient Near East*. 2 Vols. Rome: Biblical Institute Press, 1980.

Harris, R. Laird, Gleason L. Archer, and Bruce K. Waltke, eds. *Theological Wordbook of the Old Testamentt*. 2 Vols. Chicago: Moody Press, 1980.

Hendel, Ronald S. *The Epic of the Patriarch: The Jacob Cycle and the Narrative Traditions of Canaan and Israel*. Harvard Semitic Monographs, no. 42. Atlanta: Scholar Press, 1987.

Hens-Pizza, Gina. *Of Methods, Monarchs, and Meanings: A Sociorhetorical Approach to Exegesis*. Macon, GA: Mercer University Press, 1996.

Hooysma, Johanna. "Die Vergewaltigung Dinas: Auslegung von Gen. 33,18-34,31." *Texte & Kontexte* 30 (July 1986): 26-46.

Jeansonne, Sharon Pace. *The Women of Genesis: From Sarah to Potiphar's Wife*. Minneapolis: Fortress, 1990.

Jenni, Ernst, and Claus Westermann, eds. *Theologisches Handwörterbuch zum Alten Testament*. 2 Vols. Munich: Kaiser, 1971-1976.

Jost, Renate. "Von 'Huren und Heiligen': Ein sozialgeschichtlicher Beitrag." In *Feministische Hermeneutik und Erstes Tesament*, ed. Hedwig Jahnow a. o., 126-37. Stuttgart: Kohlhammer, 1994.

Kam, Rose Sallberg. *Their Stories, Our Stories: Women of the Bible*. New York: Continuum, 1995.

Kass, Leon R. "Regarding Daughters and Sisters: The Rape of Dinah." *Commentary* 93 (April 1992): 29-38.

Keefe, Alice A. "Rapes of Women/Wars of Men." *Semeia* 61 (1993): 79-94.

Kevers, Paul. "Étude litteraire de Genése 34." *Revue Biblique* 87 (January 1980): 38-86.

Klassen, William. "Love, New Testament." In *The Anchor Bible Dictionary*. Vol. 4. New York: Doubleday, 1992.

Klein, Ralph W. "Israel/Today's Believers and the Nations: Three Test Cases." *Currents in Theology and Mission* 24, no. 3 (June 1997): 232-37.

Kunin, Seth Daniel. *The Logic of Incest: A Structuralist Analysis of Hebrew Mythology*. Sheffield, UK: Sheffield Academic Press, 1995.

Lockwood, Peter L. "Jacob's Other Twin: Reading the Rape of Dinah in Context." *Lutheran Theological Journal* 29 (1995): 98-105.

Luke, K. *Studies on the Book of Genesis*. Pontifical Institute of Theology and Philosophy. Alwaye, India: Assisi Press, 1975.

Mandelkern, Solomon. *Veteris Testamenti Concordantiae Hebraicae atque Chaldaicae*. Tel Aviv: Schocken, 1967.

Marböck, J. "נבל nabal, nebalah." In *Theologisches Wörterbuch zum Alten Testament*, ed. Heinz-Josef Fabry and Helmer Ringgren, 171-186. Vol. 5. Stuttgart: Kohlhammer, 1986.

Marmesh, Ann. "Anti-Covenant." In *Anti-Covenant: Counter-Reading Women's Lives in the Hebrew Bible*, ed. Mieke Bal, 43-58. JSOT Supplement 81: Bible and Literature 22. Sheffield, UK: Almond Press, 1989.

Matthews, Victor H. and Don C. Benjamin. "Social Sciences and Biblical Studies." *Semeia:* Honor and Shame in the World of the Bible 18 (1996): 7-21.

Milgrom, Jacob. *Leviticus 1-16: A New Translation*. The Anchor Bible. New York; Doubleday, 1991.

Mitchell, Stephen. *Genesis: A New Translation of the Classic Biblical Stories*. New York: HarperCollins, 1996.

Munk, Eli. *The Call of the Torah: An Anthology of Interpretation and Commentary of the Five Books of Moses*. Translated by E. S. Mazer. New York: Mesorah, 1994.

New Interpreter's Bible: A Commentary in Twelve Volumes. Vol. 1. Nashville, TN: Abingdon, 1994.

Niditch, Susan. "The Ideology of Tricksterism." Chap. in *War in the Hebrew Bible: A Study in the Ethics of Violence*. New York: Oxford University Press, 1993.

Nielsen, Eduard. *Shechem: A Tradition-Historical Investigation*. Copenhagen: Gad, 1955.

Noble, Paul. "A 'Balanced' Reading of the Rape of Dinah: Some Exegetical and Methodological Observations." *Biblical Interpretation* 4 (1996): 173-204.

Olyan, Saul M. "Honor, Shame, and Covenant Relations in Ancient Israel and Its Environment." *Journal of Biblical Literature* 115, no. 2 (1996): 201-218.

Otto, Eckart. *Jacob in Sichem: Überlieferungsgeschichtliche, archäologische und territorialgeschichtliche Studien zur Entstehungsgeschichte Israels*. BWANT 110. Stuttgart: Kohlhammer Verlag, 1979.

Otwell, J. H. *And Sarah Laughed: The Status of Women in the Old Testament*. Philadelphia: Westminster Press, 1971.

Pedersen, Johs. "The Soul, Its Powers and Capacity." Chap. in *Israel: Its Life and Culture*. London: Cumberlege, 1926; reprint 1959.

Petermann, Ina J. "Travestie in der Exegese? Über die patriarchalische Funktionalisierung eines gynozentrischen Bibeltextes: Das Buch Ruth und seine Kommentare." *Dielheimer Blätter zum Alten Testament* 22 (1985): 74-117.

Philipps, Anthony. "NEBALAH." *Vetus Testamentum* 25 (1975): 237-41.

Pressler, Carolyn. "Sexual Violence and Deuteronomic Law." In *A Feminist Companion to Exodus to Deuteronomy*, ed. Athalya Brenner, 102-12. Sheffield, UK: Sheffield Academic Press: 1994.

————. *The View of Women Found in Deuteronomic Family Law*. BZAW. Berlin: de Gruyter, 1993.

Prewitt, Terry J. *The Elusive Covenant: A Structural-Semiotic Reading of Genesis*. Bloomington: Indiana University Press, 1990.

Prior, Michael. *The Bible and Colonialism: A Moral Critique*. Sheffield: Sheffield Academic Press, 1997.

Propp, William H. "The Origins of Infant Circumcision in Israel." *Hebrew Annual Review* 11 (1987): 355-70.

Ramras-Rauch, Gila. "Fathers and Daughters: Two Biblical Narratives (Gen 34; Judg 11)." In *Mappings of the Biblical Terrain*, ed. V. Tollers and J. Mai, 158-69. Cranbury, NJ: Associated University Presses, 1990.

Rashkow, Ilona N. *The Phallacy of Genesis: A Feminist-Psychoanalytic Approach*. Louisville, KY: Westminster and Knox Press, 1993.

Reid, Stephen Breck. *Listening In: A Multicultural Reading of the Psalms*. Nashville, TN: Abingdon Press, 1997.

Rendsburg, Gary A. *The Redaction of Genesis*. Winona Lake, IN: Eisenbrauns, 1986.

Ringgren, Helmer. *Israelitische Religion*. 2d rev. ed. Stuttgart: Kohlhammer, 1982.

Rösel, Hartmut N. *Israel in Kanaan: Zum Problem der Entstehung Israels*. Beiträge zur Erforschung des Alten Testaments und des Antiken Judentums 11. Frankfurt: Lang, 1992.

Rosenblatt, Naomi H., and Joshua Horwitz. *Wrestling with Angels: What the First Family of Genesis Teaches Us about our Spiritual Identity, Sexuality, and Personal Relationships*. New York: Delacorte, 1995.

Ruppert, Lothar. *Das Buch Genesis*. Teil II: *Kap. 25,19-50,26*. Geistliche Schriftlesung 6/2. Düsseldorf: Patmos Verlag, 1984.

Russell, Letty M., ed. *Feminist Interpretation of the Bible*. Philadelphia: Westminster Press, 1985.

Saebo, M. "נבל nabal." In *Theologisches Handwörterbuch zum Alten Testament*, ed. Ernst Jenni and Claus Westermann, 26-31. Vol. 2. Munich: Kaiser, 1976.

Sakenfeld, Katherine Doob. "Love, Old Testament." In *The Anchor Bible Dictionary*. Vol. 4. New York: Doubleday, 1992.

Sandmel, Samuel. *The Hebrew Scriptures: An Introduction to Their Literature and Religious Ideas*. New York: Oxford University Press, 1978.

Sarna, Nahum M. "The Ravishing of Dinah: A Commentary on Genesis 34." In *Studies in Jewish Education and Judaica in Honor of Louis Newman*, ed. Alexander M. Shapiro and Burton I. Cohen, 143-56. New York: Ktav, 1984.

Schmitt, Götz. "Der Ursprung des Levitentums." *Zeitschrift für die alttestamentliche Wissenschaft* 94 (1982): 575-99.

Scholder, Klaus. *The Birth of Modern Critical Theology: Origins and Problems of Biblical Criticism in the Seventeenth Century*. Translated by John Bowden. Philadelphia: Trinity Press, 1990.

Schreiner, J. "ילד jalad." In *Theologisches Wörterbuch zum Alten Testament*, ed. Heinz-Josef Fabry and Helmer Ringgren, 633-639. Vol. 3. Stuttgart: Kohlhammer, 1982.

Schulte, Hannelis. "Beobachtungen zum Begriff der Zona im Alten Testament." *Zeitschrift für die alttestamentliche Wissenschaft* 104 (1992): 255-62.

Schüssler, Elisabeth Fiorenza. "The Ethics of Interpretation: De-Centering Biblical Scholarship." *Journal of Biblical Literature* 107, no. 1 (March 1988): 3-17.

Scott, Bernard Brandon. *Hollywood Dreams and Biblical Stories.* Minneapolis: Fortress, 1994.

Scroggs, Robbin. "The Bible as Foundational Document." *Interpretation* 49, no. 1 (January 1995): 17-30.

Seale, Morris S. *The Desert Bible: Nomadic Tribal Culture and Old Testament Interpretation.* New York: St. Martin's, 1974.

Seebaß, Horst. "נפש naepaes." In *Theologisches Wörterbuch zum Alten Testament,* ed. Heinz-Josef Fabry and Helmer Ringgren, 531-555. Vol. 5. Stuttgart: Kohlhammer, 1986.

Segovia, Fernando F., and Mary Ann Tolbert, eds. *Reading from This Place.* 2 Vols. Minneapolis: Fortress, 1995.

Shapira, Amnon. "Be Silent: An Immoral Behavior?" *Beit Mikra* 39 (1994): 232-44.

Sheres, Ita. *Dinah's Rebellion: A Biblical Parable for Our Time.* New York: Crossroad, 1990.

Smith, Theophus H. *Conjuring Culture: Biblical Formations of Black America.* New York: Oxford University Press, 1994.

Smitten, Wilhelm Th. in der. "Gen 34: Ausdruck der Volksmeinung?" *Bibliotheca Orientalis* 30 (1973): 7-9.

Soggin, J. Alberto. "Genesis Kapitel 34: Eros und Thanatos." In *History and Traditions of Early Israel: Studies Presented to Eduard Nielsen,* ed. André Lemaire and Benedikt Otzen, 133-135. Leiden: Brill, 1993.

Steinmetz, Devora. *From Father to Son: Kinship, Conflict, and Continuity in Genesis.* Louisville, KY: Westminster and Knox Press, 1991.

Stendahl, Krister. "The Bible as a Classic and the Bible as Holy Scripture." *Journal of Biblical Literature* 103, no. 1 (1984): 3-10.

———. "Biblical Theology, Contemporary." *Interpreter's Dictionary of the Bible,* vol. 1 (1962): 418-32.

Sternberg, Meir. "Biblical Poetics and Sexual Politics: From Reading to Counterreading." *Journal of Biblical Literature* 111, no. 3 (1992): 463-88.

———. *The Poetics of Biblical Narrative: Ideological Literature and the Drama of Reading.* Bloomington: Indiana University Press, 1987.

Sugirtharajah, R. S., ed. *Voices from the Margin: Interpreting the Bible in the Third World.* Maryknoll: Orbis, 1991.

Thistlewaite, Susan Brooks. "'You May Enjoy the Spirit of Your Enemies': Rape as a Biblical Metaphor for War." In *Women, War,
and Metaphor: Language and Society in the Study of the
Hebrew Bible*, ed. C. V. Camp and C. R. Fontaine, 59-75. Semeia
61. Atlanta: Scholars Press, 1993.

Thibodeau, Lucille Claire. "The Relation of Peter Abelard's 'Planctus
Dinae' to Biblical Sources and Exegete Tradition: A Historical
and Textual Study." Ph. D. diss., Harvard University, 1990.

Todd, William. *New Light on Genesis: The Narrative Explained
against Its Geographical, Historical and Social Background.*
London: Furnival, 1978.

Trible, Phyllis. *Rhetorical Criticism: Context, Method, and the Book
of Jonah.* Minneapolis: Fortress, 1994.

————. *Texts of Terror.* Philadelphia: Fortress, 1984.

Vaux, Roland de. *Ancient Israel: Its Life and Institutions.* London:
Darton, 1961.

Vawter, Bruce. *On Genesis: A New Reading.* Garden City, NY:
Doubleday, 1977.

Visotzky, Burton L. *The Genesis of Ethics: How The Tormented
Family of Genesis Leads Us to Moral Development.* New York:
Crown, 1996.

Wallis, G. "חשק ḥāšaq." In *Theologisches Wörterbuch zum Alten
Testament*, ed. Heinz-Josef Fabry and Helmer Ringgren, 280-
281. Vol. 3. Stuttgart: Kohlhammer, 1982.

————. "אהב 'ahab." In *Theologisches Wörterbuch zum Alten Testament*, ed. Heinz-Josef Fabry and Helmer Ringgren, 105-128.
Vol. 1. Stuttgart: Kohlhammer, 1973.

Waltke, Bruce K., and M. O'Connor. *An Introduction to Biblical
Hebrew Syntax.* Winona Lake, Indiana: Eisenbrauns, 1990.

Weinfeld, Moshe. *The Book of Genesis.* Encyclopedia of the World of
the Tanakh. Rabibim, 1982.

————. *Deuteronomy and the Deuteronomic School.* Oxford, UK:
Clarendon Press, 1972.

West, S. A. "The Rape of Dinah and the Conquest of Shechem." *Dor
le Dor* 8 (1980): 144-57.

Whitelam, Keith. *The Invention of Ancient Israel: The Silencing of
Palestinian History.* London: Routledge, 1996.

Wilson, R. Mc. "The Early History of the Exegesis of Genesis 1,26."
In *Studia Patristica 1*, ed. Kurt Aland and F. L. Cross, 420-31.
Berlin: Akademie Verlag, 1957.

Wimbush, Vincent. "Biblical-Historical Study as Liberation: Toward an Afro-Christian Hermeneutic." *Journal of Religious Thought* 42, no. 2 (Fall-Winter 1985-1986): 9-21.

Wolff, Hans Walter. *Anthropologie des Alten Testaments.* München: Kaiser, 1977.

Wyatt, Nicolas. "The Story of Dinah and Shechem." *Ugarit-Forschungen* 22 (1990): 433-58.

Zakovitch, Y. "Assimilation in Biblical Narratives." In *Empirical Models for Biblical Criticism,* ed. Jeffrey H. Tigay, 175-96. Philadelphia: University of Pennsylvania Press, 1985.

Interdisciplinary Sources

Forensic Medical Textbooks of Nineteenth-Century Germany

Bergmann, Carl Georg Lucas Christian. *Lehrbuch der Medicina forensis für Juristen.* Braunschweig: Vieweg, 1846.

Bernt, Joseph. *Systematisches Handbuch der Staats-Arzneykunde, zum Gebrauche für Aerzte, Rechtsgelehrte, Polizeybeamte und zum Leitfaden bey öffentlichen Vorlesungen.* Erster Theil: Die öffentliche Gesundheitspflege. Vienna: Kupffer und Wimmer, 1816.

————. *Beyträge zur gerichtlichen Arzneykunde für Ärzte, Wundärzte und Rechtsgelehrte.* Erster Band. Vienna: C. Gerold, 1818.

Bocker, Friedrich Wilhelm. *Lehrbuch der gerichtlichen Medicin, mit Berücksichtigung der gesammten deutschen und rheinischen Gesetzgebung als Leitfaden zu seinen Vorlesungen und zum Gebrauche für Aerzte und Juristen.* 2. sehr vermehrte und verbesserte Auflage. Iserlohn: Badeker, 1857.

Bohn, Johann. *Dissertatio medico-legalis de phlebotomia culposa.* Lipsiae: Litteris Joh. Gottliebii Bauchii [1713].

Brach, Bernhard. *Lehrbuch der Gerichtlichen Medicin.* Cologne: F. C. Eisen, 1846.

Buchner, Ernst. *Lehrbuch der gerichtlichen Medicin für Aerzte und Juristen.* Munich: J. A. Finsterlin, 1867.

————. *Lehrbuch der gerichtlichen Medicin für Aerzte und Juristen.* 2. vermehrte und mit Rücksicht auf die deutsche Gesetzgebung umgearbeitete Auflage. Nach dem Tode des Verfassers hrsg. von C. Hecker. Munich: J. A. Finsterlin, 1872.

Casper, Johann Ludwig. *Practisches Handbuch der gerichtlichen Medicin*. Biologischer Theil. Zweiter Band. Berlin: August Hirschwald, 1858.

————. *Practisches Handbuch der Gerichtlichen Medizin*. Neu bearbeitet und vermehrt von Carl Liman. Erster Band (Biologischer Theil). 5. Auflage. Berlin: August Hirschwald, 1871.

————. *A Handbook of the Practice of Forensic Medicine, Based upon Personal Experience*. Translated from the 3rd ed. of the original by Geo. W. Balfour. 4 Vols. London: New Sydenham Society, 1861-1865.

Dittrich, Paul. *Lehrbuch der gerichtlichen Medicin für Studirende und Aerzte*. Vienna: Braumüller, 1897.

Emmert, Carl. *Lehrbuch der gerichtlichen Medizin, mit Berücksichtigung der deutschen, österreichischen und bernischen Gesetzgebungen*. Leipzig: Thieme, 1900.

Friedreich, Johannes Baptista. *Handbuch der Gerichtsaerztlichen Praxis, mit Einschluss der gerichtlichen Veterinärkunde*. 2 Bände. Regensburg: G. J. Munz, 1843-1844.

Guder, Paul. *Gerichtliche Medizin für Mediziner und Juristen*. 2. Auflage, unter Berücksichtigung des Bürgerlichen Gesetzbuches, des Unfall-Versicherungs- und des Alters- und Invaliditäts-Versicherungs-Gesetzes, bearb. von Paul Stolper. Leipzig: Barth, 1900.

Güntner, Franz Xaver. *Handbuch der gerichtlichen Medizin für Mediziner, Rechtsgelehrte und Gerichtsärzte, mit Rücksichtnahme auf die Schwurgerichte*. Regensburg: Manz, 1851.

Hauska, Ferdinand. *Compendium der gerichtlichen Arzneikunde*. 2. umgearbeitete Auflage. Vienna: Braumüller, 1869.

Henke, Adolph Christian Heinrich. *Lehrbuch der gerichtlichen Medicin: Zum Behufe academischer Vorlesungen und zum Gebrauch für gerichtliche Ärzte und Rechtsgelehrte entworfen*. Berlin: J. E. Hitzig, 1812.

————. *Lehrbuch der gerichtlichen Medicin: Zum Behufe academischer Vorlesungen und zum Gebrauch für gerichtliche Ärzte und Rechtsgelehrte entworfen*. 13. Auflage mit Nachträgen von Carl Bergmann. Berlin: Ferdinand Dümmler, 1859.

Hofmann, Eduard, Ritter von. *Lehrbuch der Gerichtlichen Medicin; mit besonderer Berücksichtigung der österreichischen und deutschen Gesetzgebung*. Vienna: Urban & Schwarzenberg, 1878.

————. *Lehrbuch der Gerichtlichen Medizin mit gleichmässiger Berücksichtigung der deutschen und österreichischen Gesetzgebung*. 3. vermehrte und verbesserte Auflage. Erste Hälfte. Vienna and Leipzig: Urban & Schwarzenberg, 1883.

————. 9. vermehrte und verbessert Auflage. Ed. Dr. Alexander Kolisko. Berlin/Vienna: Urban & Schwarzenberg, 1903.

Klose, Wolfgang Friedrich Wilhelm. *System der gerichtlichen Physik*. Breslau: Johann Friedrich Korn, 1814.

————. *Beyträge zur gerichtlichen Arzneikunde*. Breslau and Leipzig: Wilhelm Gottlieb Korn, 1811.

Kornfeld, Hermann. *Handbuch der gerichtlichen Medicin in Beziehung zu der Gesetzgebung Deutschlands und des Auslandes, nebst einem Anhange enthaltend die einschlägigen Gesetze und Verordnungen Deutschlands, Oesterreichs und Frankreichs*. Stuttgart: Ferdinand Enke, 1884.

Kramer, Friedrich Ludwig. *Handbuch der gerichtlichen Medizin, für Aerzte und Juristen*. 2., umgearbeitete Auflage. Braunschweig: C. A. Schwetschke, 1857.

Lion, Adolph. *Taschenbuch der gerichtlichen Medicin nach dem neuesten Standpunkt der Wissenschaft und der Gesetzgebungen Deutschlands zum Gebrauche für Aerzte und Juristen*. Erlangen: Ferdinand Enke, 1861.

Maschka, J., ed. *Handbuch der Gerichtlichen Medicin*. 3. Band. Tübingen: H. Laupp, 1882.

Masius, Georg Heinrich. *System der gerichtlichen Arzneykunde für Rechtsgelehrte*. Rostock: Altona, 1810.

————. *Lehrbuch der gerichtlichen Arzneikunde für Rechtsgelehrte*. Zweiter Theil. 2., sehr vermehrte und verbesserte Ausgabe. Altona: Johann Friedrich Hammerich, 1812.

————. *Handbuch der gerichtlichen Arzneiwissenschaft. Zum Gebrauche für gerichtliche Ärzte und Rechtsgelehrte*. Erster Band. Erste Abtheilung. 3. Ausgabe. Stendal: Franzen und Grosse, 1821.

Meckel, August Albert. *Lehrbuch der gerichtlichen Medicin*. Halle: C. F. Schimmelpfennig, 1821.

Mende, Ludwig Julius Kaspar. *Ausführliches Handbuch der gerichtlichen Medizin für Gesetzgeber, Rechtsgelehrte, Aerzte und Wundärzte*. 4. Band. Leipzig: Onk'sche Buchhandlung, 1826.

Metzger, Johann Daniel. *Kurzgefasstes System der gerichtlichen Arzneywissenschaft.* Nach dem Todte des Verfassers revidirt, verbessert, mit den nöthigen Zusätzen und einem Register versehen von Dr. Christian Gottfried Gruner. 4. verbesserte und vermehrte Ausgabe. Königsberg/Leipzig: August Wilhelm Unzer, 1814.

————. *System der gerichtlichen Arzneywissenschaft.* Nach dem Tode des Verfassers verbessert und mit Zusätzen versehen von Dr. Christian Gottfried Gruner. Erweitert und berichtigt von Wilhelm Hermann Georg Remer. 5. Auflage. Königsberg/Leipzig: August Wilhelm Unzer, 1820.

————. *Handbuch der Staatsarzneykunde, enthaltend die medicinische Policey und gerichtliche Arzneywissenschaft.* Züllichau: R. G. Fromanns, 1787.

Michaelis, Adolph Albert. *Systema jurisprudentiae medicae.*VI. Tom. 4 tom. Halle 1725-1736.

Müller, Johann Valentin. *Entwurf der gerichtlichen Arzneywissenschaft nach juristischen und medicinischen Grundsätzen, für Geistliche, Rechtsgelehrte und Aerzte.* Vol. I. Frankfurt am Main: Andreäische Buchhandlung, 1796.

Ney, Franz von. *Systematisches Handbuch der gerichtsarzneilichen Wissenschaft mit besonderer Berücksichtigung der Erhebung des Thatbestandes im Straf- und Civilverfahren für Aerzte, Wundärzte, dann Justiz- und politische Beamte und Advokaten in den k.k. Staaten, nebst einem Anhange über den Geschäfststyl.* Vienna: Mörschner's Witwe & W. Bianchi, 1845.

Nicolai, Johann August Heinrich. *Handbuch der gerichtlichen Medicin nach dem gegenwärtigen Standpunkt dieser Wissenschaft für Aerzte und Criminalisten.* Berlin: August Hirschwald, 1841.

Niemann, Johann Friedrich. *Handbuch der Staats-Arzneywissenschaft und staatsärztlichen Veterinärkunde nach alphabetischer Ordnung für Aerzte, Medicinalpolizei-Beamte und Richter.* 2 Bände. Leipzig: Johann Ambrosius Barth, 1813.

Pichler, Wilhelm. *Die gerichtliche Medizin, nach dem heutigen Standpunkte der Medizin und der Gesetzgebung in ihren Umrissen dargestellt.* Vienna: Wallishausser, 1861.

Roose, Theodor Georg August. *Grundriss medizinisch-gerichtlicher Vorlesungen.* Frankfurt am Main: Wilmans, 1802.

Schauenstein, Adolf. *Lehrbuch der gerichtlichen Medizin, mit besonderer Berücksichtigung der Gesetzgebung Oesterreichs und deren Vergleichung mit den Gesetzgebungen Deutschlands, Frankreichs und Englands, für Aerzte und Juristen.* Vienna: Braunmüller, 1862.

Schmidtmann, A., ed. *Handbuch der Gerichtlichen Medizin.* 9. Auflage des Casper-Liman'schen Handbuches. 1. Band. Berlin: Verlag von August Hirschwald, 1905.

Schmidtmüller, Johann Anton. *Handbuch der Staatsarzneykunde zu Vorlesungen und zum Gebrauche für Bezirksärzte, Polizei- und Justizbeamte.* Landshut: Krüll, 1804.

Schürmayer, Ignaz Heinrich. *Theoretisch-practisches Lehrbuch der Gerichtlichen Medicin: Mit Berücksichtigung der neueren Gesetzgebungen des In- und Auslandes und des Verfahrens bei Schwurgerichten, für Ärzte und Juristen: Mit einem Anhange, enthaltend eine kurzgefasste practische Anleitung zu gerichtlichen Leichenobductionen.* Erlangen: Ferdinand Enke, 1850.

————. *Lehrbuch der Gerichtlichen Medicin: Mit Berücksichtigung der neueren Gesetzgebungen des In- und Auslandes insbesondere des Verfahrens bei Schwurgerichten. Für Ärzte und Juristen. Mit einem Anhange.* 2. Auflage. Erlangen: Ferdinand Enke, 1854.

————. *Lehrbuch der Gerichtlichen Medicin: Mit Berücksichtigung der neueren Gesetzgebungen des In- und Auslandes insbesondere des Verfahrens bei Schwurgerichten. Für Ärzte und Juristen. Mit einem Anhange.* 3. gänzlich umgearbeitete und verbesserte Auflage. Erlangen: Ferdinand Enke, 1861.

————. *Lehrbuch der Gerichtlichen Medicin: Mit vorzüglicher Berücksichtigung des deutschen Strafgesetzbuches. Für Äerzte und Juristen.* 4. verbesserte und vermehrte Auflage. Erlangen: Ferdinand Enke, 1874.

Siebenhaar, Friedrich Julius. *Enzyklopädisches Handbuch der gerichtlichen Arzneikunde für Aerzte und Rechtsgelehrte.* In Verbindung mit Friedr. Erdm. Flachs et al. 2 Bände. Leipzig: Engelmann, 1838-1840.

Siebold, Casper Jacob von. *Lehrbuch der gerichtlichen Medicin: Zur Grundlage bei academischen Vorlesungen und zum Gebrauch für gerichtliche Aerzte und Rechtsgelehrte.* Berlin: Theod. Chr. Fr. Enslin, 1847.

Strassmann, Fritz. *Lehrbuch der gerichtlichen Medicin*. Mit 78 in den Text eingedruckten Abbildungen und einer Tafel in Farbendruck. Stuttgart: Ferdinand Enke, 1895.

Wildberg, Christian Friedrich Ludwig. *Handbuch der gerichtlichen Arzneywissenschaft zur Grundlage bey akademischen Vorlesungen und zum Gebrauche für ausübende gerichtliche Aerzte*. Berlin: W. Dieterici, 1812.

————. *Lehrbuch der gerichtlichen Arzneiwissenschaft: Zum Gebrauch academischer Vorlesungen*. Erfurt: Keyser, 1824.

————. *Entwurf eines Codex Medico Forensis, oder Zusammenstellung der bei Ausübung der gerichtlichen Arzneiwissenschaft allgemein zu befolgenden Vorschriften*. Berlin: Schlesinger, 1842.

————. *Codex Medico-Forensis, oder Inbegriff aller in gerichtlichen Fällen von den Gerichts-Aerzten zu beobachtender Vorschriften*. Neu bearbeitet. Leipzig: F. A. Brockhaus, 1849.

History of Forensic Medicine

Ackerknecht, Erwin H. "Legal Medicine in Transition (16th-18th Centuries)." *Ciba Symposia* 11, no. 7 (Winter 1950-1951): 1290-98.

————. "Legal Medicine Becomes a Modern Science (19th Century)." *Ciba Symposia* 11, no. 7 (Winter 1950-1951): 1299-1304.

Brittain, Robert P. "Origins of Legal Medicine: Constitution Criminalis Carolina." *Medicolegal Journal* 33 (1965): 124-27.

Clark, Michael and Catherine Crawford, eds. *Legal Medicine in History*. Cambridge, UK: Cambridge University Press, 1994.

Crawford, Catherine. "Medicine and the Law." In *Encyclopedia of the History of Medicine*, ed. W. F. Bynum and Roy Porter, 1619-40. Vol. 2. London/New York: Routledge, 1993.

Curran, William J. "The Confusion of Titles in the Medicolegal Field: An Historical Analysis and a Proposal for Reform." *Medicine, Science and the Law* 15 (1975): 270-75.

Davis, B. "A History of Forensic Medicine." *Medicolegal Journal* 53 (1985): 9-23.

Fischer-Homberger, Esther. *Medizin vor Gericht: Gerichtsmedizin von der Renaissance bis zur Aufklärung*. Bern: Verlag Hans Huber, 1983.

Miller, Dr. "Ueber Nothzucht." *Adolph Henke's Zeitschrift für die Staatsarzneikunde* 54B (1847): 249-92.

Meyer-Knees, Anke. *Verführung und sexuelle Gewalt: Untersuchung zum medizinischen und juristischen Diskurs im 18. Jahrhundert.* Probleme der Semiotik. Vol. 12. Tübingen: Stauffenburg, 1992.

Myers, Richard O. "Famous Forensic Scientists: 7-Eduard Ritter von Hofmann (1837-1897)." *Medicine, Science and the Law* 3, no. 1 (October 1962): 18-24.

Nemec, Jaroslav. *Highlights in Medicolegal Relations.* Rev. and enlarged ed. Bethesda, MD: U.S. Department of Health, Education and Welfare, 1976.

Placzek, S. "Geschichte der gerichtlichen Medizin." In *Handbuch der Geschichte der Medizin,* ed. Max Neuburger and Julius Pagel, 729-66. Vol. 3. Jena: Gustav Fischer, 1905.

Reuter, Fritz. *Geschichte der Wiener Lehrkanzel für gerichtliche Medizin von 1804-1954.* Beiträge zur Gerichtlichen Medizin. XIX Supplement. Vienna: Franz Deuticke, 1954.

Schönbauer, Leopold. *Das Medizinische Wien: Geschichte, Werden, Würdigung.* 2. umgearbeitete und erweiterte Auflage. Vienna: Urban & Schwarzenberg, 1947.

Smith, Syndey Alfred. "The History and Development of Legal Medicine." In *Legal Medicine,* ed. R. B. H. Gradwohl, 1-19. St. Louis: Mosby, 1954.

Teufert Eveline. *Notzucht und sexuelle Nötigung: Ein Beitrag zur Kriminologie und Kriminalistik der Sexualfreiheitsdelikte unter Berücksichtigung der Geschichte und der geltenden strafrechtlichen Regelung.* Kriminalwissenschaftliche Abhandlungen. Band 14. Lübeck: Max Schmidt-Römhild, 1980.

Weeks, Jeffrey. "Sexuality and the Historian." Chap. in *Sex, Politics and Society: The Regulation of Sexuality since 1800.* London: Longman, 1981.

Feminist Scholarship on Rape since the 1970s

Adams, Carol J. and Marie Fortune, eds. *Violence against Women and Children: A Christian Theological Sourcebook.* New York: Continuum, 1995.

Adisa, Opal Palmer. "Undeclared War: African-American Writers Explicating Rape." *Women's Studies Forum* 15, no. 3 (1992): 363-74.

Agnes, Flavia. "The Anti-Rape Campaign: The Struggle and the Setback." In *The Struggle against Violence,* ed. Chhaya Datar, 99-150. Calcutta: Stree, 1993.

Alexander, Cheryl S. "The Responsible Victim: Nurses' Perceptions of Victims of Rape." *Journal of Health and Social Behavior* 21, no. 1 (March 1980): 22-33.

Allison, Julie A. *Rape: The Misunderstood Crime.* Newbury Park, CA: Sage, 1993.

Aptheker, Bettina. *Woman's Legacy: Essays on Race, Sex, and Class in American History.* Amherst: University of Massachusetts, 1982.

Armstrong, A. *Women and Rape in Zimbabwe.* Human & People's Right Project. Monograph No. 10. Lesotho: Institute of Southern African Studies, 1990.

Bart, Pauline B. "Rape as a Paradigm of Sexism in Society: Victimization and Its Discontents." *Women's Studies International Quarterly* 2 (1979): 347-57.

Bechhofer, Laurie, and Andrea Parrot. "What Is Acquaintance Rape?" In *Acquaintance Rape: The Hidden Crime,* ed. Andrea Parrot and Laurie Bechhofer, 9-25. New York: Wiley, 1991.

Bell, Diane. "Interracial Rape Revisited: On Forging a Feminist Future beyond Factions and Frightening Politics." *Women's Studies International Forum* 14 (1991): 385-412.

————, and Topsy Napurrula Nelson. "Speaking about Rape Is Everyone's Business." *Women's Studies International Forum* 12, no. 4 (1989): 403-16.

Blakely, Mary Kay. "The New Bedford Verdict: Did It Really Change Our Thinking about Rape?" *MS.* 13 (July 1984): 116.

Bounds, Elizabeth M. "Sexuality and Economic Reality: A First World and Third World Comparison." In *Redefining Sexual Ethics: A Sourcebook of Essays, Stories, and Poems,* ed. Susan E. Davies and Eleanor H. Haney, 131-143. Cleveland: Pilgrim Press, 1991.

"Branch of National Union of Journalists Proposes Guidelines on Rape Reporting." *Media Report to Women* 11, no. 4 (July-August 1983): 3, 12, 13.

Brewer, James D. *The Danger from Strangers: Confronting the Threat of Assault.* New York: Plenum, 1994.

Bridges, Judith S., and Christine A. McGrail. "Attributions of Responsibility for Date and Stranger Rape." *Sex Roles* 21, no. 3-4 (1989): 273-86.

Brownmiller, Susan. *Against Our Will: Men, Women and Rape.* New York: Bantam, 1975.

Carby, Hazel. "On the Threshold of Woman's Era: Lynching, Empire, and Sexuality in Black Feminist Theory." *Critical Inquiry* 12 (Autumn 1985): 262-77.

Check, James V. P., and Neil M. Malamuth. "Sex Role Stereotyping and Reactions to Depictions of Stranger versus Acquaintance Rape." *Journal of Personality and Social Psychology* 45, no. 2 (1983): 344-56.

Collins, Patricia. *Black Feminist Thought: Knowledge, Consciousness, and the Politics of Empowerment.* New York: Routledge, 1990.

Crenshaw, Kimberlé Williams. "Mapping the Margins: Intersectionality, Identity Politics, and Violence against Women of Color." In *The Public Nature of Private Violence: The Discovery of Domestic Abuse,* ed. Martha Albertson Fineman and Roxanne Mykitiuk, 93-118. New York/London: Routledge, 1994.

Curtis, Lynn A. "Rape, Race, and Culture: Some Speculations in Search of a Theory." In *Sexual Assault: The Victim and the Rapist,* ed. Marcia J. Walker and Stanley L. Brodsky, 117-34. Toronto/London: Heath, 1976.

Davis, Angela Y. *Violence against Women and the Ongoing Challenge to Racism.* 1st ed. Freedom Organizing Series. Latham, NY: Kitchen Table, Women of Color Press, 1991.

———. *Women, Race & Class.* New York: Random House, 1981.

———. "Rape, Racism and the Capitalist Setting." *Black Scholar* 9, no. 7 (1978): 24-30.

Denmark, Florence L., and Susan B. Friedman. "Social Psychological Aspects of Rape." In *Violence against Women: A Critique of the Sociobiology of Rape,* ed. Suzanne R. Sunday and Ethel Tobach, 159-84. New York: Gordian Press, 1985.

Dworkin, Andrea. *Intercourse.* New York: Free Press, 1987.

Estrich, Susan. *Real Rape.* Cambridge, MA: Harvard University Press, 1987.

Feild, Hubert S. "Attitudes toward Rape: A Comparative Analysis of Police, Rapists, Crisis Counselor and Citizens." *Journal of Personality and Social Psychology* 36 (1978): 156-79.

Foe, Pamela. "What's Wrong with Rape." In *Feminism and Philosophy,* ed. Mary Vetterling-Braggin, Frederick A. Elliston, and Jane English, 347-59. Totowa, NJ: Littlefield, Adams, 1981.

Fortune, Marie M. *Love Does Not Harm: Sexual Ethics For the Rest of Us.* New York: Continuum, 1995.

Fout, John C. "The Woman's Role in the German Working-Class Family in the 1890s from the Perspective of Women's Autobiographies." In *German Women in the Nineteenth Century: A Social History,* ed. John C. Fout, 295-19. New York: Holmes & Meier, 1984.

Funk, Rus Erwin. *Stopping Rape: A Challenge for Men.* Philadelphia: New Society, 1993.

Gager, Nancy, and Cathleen Schurr. *Sexual Assault: Confronting Rape in America.* New York: Grosset & Dunlap, 1976.

Gamble, Nancy C., and Lee Madigan. *The Second Rape: Society's Continued Betrayal of the Victim.* New York: Lexington, 1991.

Ginsberg, Elaine, and Sara Lennox. "Antifeminism in Scholarship and Publishing." In *Antifeminism in the Academy,* ed. VéVé Clark a.o., 169-99 New York: Routledge, 1996.

Gnanadason, Aruna. "Violence against Women: Women against Violence." Unpublished Paper for a Conference at Rochester Divinity School, November 9-13, 1995.

Gordon, Margaret, and Stephanie Riger. *The Female Fear.* New York: Free Press, 1989.

Gravdal, Kathryn. *Ravishing Maidens: Writing Rape in Medieval French Literature and Law.* Philadelphia: University of Pennsylvania Press, 1991.

Griffin, Susan. *Rape: The Power of Consciousness.* New York: Harper & Row, 1979.

———. "Rape: The All-American Crime." *Ramparts* (1971): 26-35.

Grossmann, Atina. "A Question of Silence: The Rape of German Women by Occupation Soldiers." *October* 72 (Spring 1995): 43-63.

Gunn, Rita, and Candice Minch. "Unofficial and Official Responses to Sexual Assault." *Resources for Feminist Research* 14 (December 1985-January 1986): 47-49.

Hall, Jacquelyn Dowd. "'The Mind That Burns in Each Body': Women, Rape, and Racial Violence." In *Powers of Desire: The Politics of Sexuality,* ed. Ann Snitow, Christine Stansell, and Sharon Thompson, 328-49. New York: Monthly Review Press, 1983.

Harding, Sandra. "The Instability of the Analytical Categories of Feminist Theory." *Signs* 11, no. 4 (1986): 645-64.

Hare-Mustin, Rachel T., and Jeanne Marecek. "Gender and the Meaning of Difference: Postmodernism and Psychology." In *Making a Difference: Psychology and the Construction of Gender,* ed. Rachel T. Hare-Mustin and Jeanne Marecek, 22-64. New Haven: Yale University Press, 1990.

Hekman, Susan. "Truth and Method: Feminist Standpoint Theory Revisited." *Signs* 22, no. 2 (Winter 1997): 341-65.

Held, Jane. "The British Peace Movement: A Critical Examination of Attitudes to Male Violence within the British Peace Movement, as Expressed with Regard to the 'Molesworth Rapes.'" *Women's Studies International Forum* 11, no. 3 (1988): 211-21.

Higgins, Lynn A., and Brenda R. Silver, eds. *Rape and Representation.* New York: Columbia University Press, 1991.

Hine, Darlene Clark. "Rape and the Inner Lives of Black Women in the Middle West: Preliminary Thoughts on the Culture of Dissemblance." *Signs* 14, no. 4 (1989): 912-20.

hooks, bell. *Yearning: Race, Gender, and Cultural Politics.* Boston: South End Press, 1990.

————. *Feminist Theory: From Margin to Center.* Boston: South End Press, 1984.

James, Stanlie M., and Abena P. A. Busia, eds. *Theorizing Black Feminisms: The Visionary Pragmatism of Black Women.* New York: Routledge: 1993.

Johnson, James D., and Lee A. Jackson. "Assessing the Effects of Factors That Might Underlie the Differential Perception of Acquaintance and Stranger Rape." *Sex Roles* 10, no. 1-2 (1988): 37-45.

Kalven, Harry, and Hans Zeisel. *The American Jury.* Boston: Little, Brown, 1966.

Kelly, Liz. "The Continuum of Sexual Violence." In *Women, Violence and Social Control,* ed. Jalna Hanmer and Mary Maynard, 46-60. Houndmills, UK: Macmillan, 1987.

Krishna, K. P. "Rapes and Its Victims in India." *Journal of Social and Economic Studies* 10 (1982): 89-100.

Kumar, Radha. "The Agitation Against Rape." Chap. in *The History of Doing: An Illustrated Account of Movements for Women's Rights and Feminism in India, 1800-1990.* London: Verso, 1990.

Larson-Thorisch, Alexa Kay. "Was It Rape? Sexual Violence and the Construction of Gender in Legal-Medical and Literary Discourse (1770-1810)." Ph.D. diss., University of Wisconsin-Madison, 1994.

Lauretis, Teresa de. "The Violence of Rhetoric: Considerations on Representation and Gender." Chap. in *Technologies of Gender: Essays on Theory, Film, and Fiction.* Bloomington/Indianapolis: Indiana University Press, 1987.

Lisak, David. "Sexual Aggression, Masculinity, and Fathers." *Signs* 16 (Winter 1991): 238-62.

Maboe, Matlhogonolo. "Strategies to Tackle Rape and Violence against Women in South Africa." In *Gender Violence and Women's*

Human Rights in Africa, ed. Center for Women's Leadership, 30-37. Highland, NJ: Plowshares, 1994.

MacKinnon, Catherine. "Sex and Violence: A Perspective." In *Rape and Society: Readings on the Problem of Sexual Assault*, ed. Patricia Searles and Ronald J. Berger, 28-34. Boulder, CO: Westview Press, 1995.

————. *Towards a Theory of the State*. Cambridge, MA: Harvard University Press, 1989.

Marcus, Sharon. "Fighting Bodies, Fighting Words: A Theory and Politics of Rape Prevention." In *Feminists Theorize the Political*, ed. Judith Butler and Joan W. Scott, 385-403. New York: Routledge, 1992.

Matoesian, Gregory M. *Reproducing Rape: Domination through Talk in the Courtroom*. Chicago: University of Chicago Press, 1993.

McGlashan, Beth. "Women Should Decide for Themselves If They Want Rape Known." *Media Report to Women* 10, no. 6 (June 1, 1982): 10-11.

Medea, Andra, and Kathleen Thompson. *Against Rape*. New York: Farrar, Straus & Giroux, 1974.

Mohanty, Chandra Talpade. "Under Western Eyes: Feminist Scholarship and Colonial Discourses." In *Third World Women and the Politics of Feminism*, ed. Ch. T. Mohanty, Ann Russo, and Lourdes Torres, 51-80. Bloomington: Indiana University Press, 1991.

National Victim Center and Crime Victims Research and Treatment Center. *Rape in America: A Report to the Nation*. April 23, 1992.

Natta, Don van. "Facts, Lies and Opinions on Trial in Unusual Sidelight to Rape Case." *New York Times* (29 January 1996): B1, B2.

Omvedt, Gail. *Violence against Women: New Movements and New Theories in India*. New Delhi: Interpress, 1990.

Pineau, Lois. "Date-Rape: A Feminist Analysis." *Law and Philosophy* 8, no. 2 (August 1989): 217-43.

Plaza, Monique. "Our Damages and Their Compensation: Rape: The Will Not to Know of Michel Foucault." *Feminist Issues* (Summer 1981): 25-35.

Rape in Malaysia: The Victims and the Rapists: The Myths and the Realities: What Can Be Done. Consumers' Association of Penang: Penang, Malaysia, 1988.

Riger, Stephanie, and Margaret T. Gordon. "The Fear of Rape: A Study in Social Control." *Journal of Social Issues* 37, no. 4 (1981): 71-92.

Rise, Eric W. "Race, Rape, and Radicalism: The Case of the Martinsville Seven, 1949-1951." *Journal of Southern History* 58, no. 3 (August 1992): 461-90.

Roberts, Cathy. *Women and Rape*. New York: New York University Press, 1989.

Rozeé, Patricia D. "Forbidden or Forgiven? Rape in Cross-Cultural Perspective." *Psychology of Women Quarterly* 17 (1993): 499-514.

Rushing, Andrea Benton. "Surviving Rape: A Morning/Mourning Ritual." In *Theorizing Black Feminisms: The Visionary Pragmatism of Black Women*, ed. Stanlie M. James and Abena P. A. Busia, 127-40. New York: Routledge, 1993.

Russel, Diana E. H. *The Politics of Rape: The Victim's Perspective*. New York: Stein and Day, 1984.

Ryan, Kathryn M. "Rape and Seduction Scripts." *Psychology of Women Quarterly* 12 (1988): 237-45.

Sanday, Peggy Reeves. *Fraternity Gang Rape: Sex, Brotherhood, and Privilege on Campus*. New York: New York University Press, 1990.

———. "The Socio-Cultural Context of Rape: A Cross-Cultural Study." *The Journal of Social Issues* 37, no. 4 (1981): 5-27.

Sander, Helke, and Roger Willemsen. *Gewaltakte, Männerphantasien & Krieg*. Hamburg: Ingrid Klein, 1993.

———, and Barbara Johr, eds. *BeFreier und Befreite: Krieg, Vergewaltigungen, Kinder*. Munich: Kunstmann, 1992.

Sanders, William B. *Rape and Woman's Identity*. Beverly Hills, CA: Sage, 1980.

Schrink, Jeffrey, Eric D. Poole, and Robert M. Regoli. "Sexual Myths and Ridicule: A Content Analysis of Rape Jokes." *Psychology: A Quarterly Journal of Human Behavior* 19, no. 1 (1982): 1-6.

Schüssler, Elisabeth Fiorenza, and Mary Shawn Copeland, eds. *Violence Against Women*. London, SCM Press, 1994.

Sharpe, Jenny. "The Unspeakable Limits of Rape: Colonial Violence and Counter-Insurgency." *Genders* 10 (Spring 1991): 25-46.

Shotland, R. Lance. "A Theory of the Causes of Courtship Rape: Part 2." *Journal of Social Issues* 48, no. 1 (1992): 127-43.

Smart, Carol. *Law, Crime and Sexuality: Essays in Feminism.* London: Sage, 1995.

Solomon, Alison. "Congress on Rape: Jerusalem, April 7-10, 1986." *Women's Studies International Forum* 9, no. 3 (1986): i-iii.

Spelman, Elizabeth V. *Inessential Women: Problems of Exclusion in Feminist Thought.* Boston: Beacon, 1988.

Tanner, Laura E. *Intimate Violence: Reading Rape and Torture in Twentieth-Century Fiction.* Bloomington: Indiana University Press, 1994.

Tetreault, Patricia A., and Mark A. Barnett. "Reactions to Stranger and Acquaintance Rape." *Psychology of Women Quarterly* 11 (1987): 353-58.

Thornton, Bill, and Richard M. Ryckman. "The Influence of a Rape Victim's Physical Attractiveness on Observers' Attributions of Responsibility." *Human Relations* 36, no. 6 (1983): 549-62.

Tomselli, Sylvana, and Roy Porter, eds. *Rape.* New York: Basil Blackwell, 1986.

Truong, Thanh-dam. *Sex, Money, and Morality: Prostitution and Tourism in South-East Asia.* London: Zed Books, 1990.

Villemur, Nora K., and Janet Shibley Hyde. "Effects of Sex of Defense Attorney, Sex of Juror, and Age and Attractiveness of the Victim on Mock Juror Decision Making in a Rape Case." *Sex Roles* 9, no. 8 (1983): 879-89.

Ward, Colleen A. *Attitudes toward Rape: Feminist and Social Psychological Perspectives.* London: Sage, 1995.

Williams, Joyce E. "Secondary Victimization: Confronting Public Attitudes about Rape." *Victimology: An International Journal* 9, no. 1 (1984): 66-81.

———, and Karen A. Holmes. *The Second Assault: Rape and Public Attitudes.* Westport, CN: Greenwood, 1981.

Williams, Lynora. "Violence against Women." *Black Scholar* (January-February 1981): 18-24.

Wilson, Wayne. "Rape as Entertainment." *Psychological Reports* 63 (1988): 607-10.

Woodhull, Winifred. "Sexuality, Power, and the Question of Rape." In *Feminism and Foucault: Reflections on Resistance,* ed. Irene Diamond and Lee Quinby, 167-76. Boston: Northeastern University Press, 1988.

Wriggins, Jennifer. "Rape, Racism, and the Law." In *Rape and Society: Readings on the Problem of Sexual Assault,* ed. Patricia Searles and Ronald J. Berger. Boulder, CO: Westview, 1995.

Other Works

Amnesty International. *Bosnia-Herzegovina: Rape and Sexual Abuse by Armed Forces*. New York: Amnesty International, 1993.

Armstrong, Paul B. *Conflicting Readings: Variety and Validity in Interpretation*. Chapel Hill: University of North Carolina Press, 1990.

Bordo, Susan. "Feminism, Postmodernism, and Gender-Scepticism." In *Feminism/Postmdernism*, ed. and with an introduction by Linda J. Nicholson, 133-56. New York: Routledge, 1990.

Bottigheimer, Ruth B. *The Bible for Children: From the Age of Gutenberg to the Present*. New Haven: Yale University Press, 1996.

Butler, Judith *Gender Trouble: Feminism and the Subversion of Identity*. New York, London: Routledge, 1990.

———. "Imitation and Gender Insubordination." Chap. in *inside/out: Lesbian Theories, Gay Theories*, ed. Diana Fuss, 13-31. New York: Routledge, 1991.

Foucault, Michel. *The History of Sexuality*. Vol. 1: *An Introduction*. Translated by Robert Hurley. New York: Vintage Books, 1990.

———. *The History of Sexuality*. Vol. 1: *An Introduction*. Translated by Robert Hurley. New York: Random House, 1978.

———. *The Archaelogy of Knowledge and the Discourse on Language*. Translated by A. M. Sherican Smith. New York: Pantheon, 1972.

Fulkerson, Mary McClintock. *Changing the Subject: Women's Discourse and Feminist Theology*. Minneapolis: Fortress, 1994.

Gadamer, Hans-Georg. *Truth and Method*. New York: Seabury Press, 1975.

Glare, P. G. W., ed. *Oxford Latin Dictionary*. 3 Vols. Oxford, UK: Clarendon Press, 1968-80.

Godard, Barbara. "Intertextuality." In *Encyclopedia of Contemporary Literary Theory: Approaches, Scholars, Terms*, ed. Irena R. Makaryk, 568-72. Toronto: University of Toronto Press, 1993.

Goold, G. P., ed. *Theaetetus, Plato*. English translation by H. North Fowler. Cambridge, MA: Harvard University Press, 1921.

Gribbin, John. *Schrödinger's Kitten and the Search for Reality: Solving the Quantum Mysteries*. Boston: Little, Brown, 1995.

Groden, Michael, and Martin Kreiswirth, eds. *The John Hopkins Guide to Literary Theory & Criticism*. Baltimore: Johns Hopkins University Press, 1994.

Grondin, Jean. "Hermeneutics and Relativism." In *Festivals of Inter-pretation: Essays on Hans-Georg Gadamer's Work*, ed. Kathleen Wright, 42-62. Albany: State University of New York Press, 1990.

Haraway, Donna J. "Situated Knowledges: The Science Question in Feminism and the Privilege of Partial Perspective." Chap. in *Simians, Cyborgs, and Women: The Reinvention of Nature*, 183-201. New York: Routledge, 1991.

Harding, Sandra. *Whose Science? Whose Knowledge? Thinking from Women's Lives*. Ithaca, NY: Cornell University Press, 1991.

Hawkesworth, Mary E. Knowers. "Knowing, Known: Feminist Theory and Claims of Truth." *Signs* 14, no. 3 (1989): 533-57.

Hoff, Joan. "Gender as a Postmodern Category of Paralysis." *Women's History Review* 3 (1994):149-68.

———. "A Reply to My Critics." *Women's History Review* 5, no. 1 (1996): 25-30.

"Justice in Peru: Victim Gets Rapist for a Husband." *New York Times* (March 12, 1997): A1, A12:

Kent, Susan Kingsley. "Mistrials and Diatribulations: A Reply to Joan Hoff." *Women's History Review* 5, no. 1 (1996): 9-18.

Leitch, Vincent B. *Cultural Criticism, Literary Theory, Post-structuralism*. New York: Columbia University Press, 1992.

———. *American Literary Criticism from the Thirties to the Eigthies*. New York: Columbia University Press, 1988.

Lentricchia, Frank, and Thomas McLaughlin, eds. *Critical Terms for Literary Study*. Chicago: University of Chicago Press, 1995.

Loewenstein, Andrea Freud. *Loathsome Jews and Engulfing Women: Metaphors of Projection in the Works of Wyndham Lewis, Charles Williams, and Graham Greene*. New York: New York University Press, 1993.

McKee, James B. *Sociology and the Race Problem: The Failure of a Perspective*. Chicago: University of Illinois Press, 1993.

Nicholson, Linda J. *Feminism/Postmodernism*. New York: Routledge, 1990.

Oxford Companion to Philosophy, 1995 ed., s.v. "Cave, analogy of," "Forms, Platonic," "Plato."

Ramazanoglu, Caroline. "Unravelling Postmodern Paralysis: A Response to Joan Hoff." *Women's History Review* 5, no. 1 (1996): 19-23.

Ricoeur, Paul. *Interpretation Theory*. Fort Worth: Texas Christian
    University Press, 1976.
Roget's International Thesaurus, rev. Robert L. Chapman. 4th ed.
    New York: HarperCollins, 1977.
Rorty, Richard. *Philosophy and the Mirror of Nature*. Princeton,
    NJ: Princeton University Press, 1979.
Ross, David. *Plato's Theory of Ideas*. Oxford, UK: Oxford University
    Press, 1951.
Said, Edward W. *Culture and Imperialism*. New York: Knopf, 1993.
———. *Orientalism*. New York: Random House, 1978.
Taylor, Gary. *Cultural Selection*. New York: Basic Books, 1996.

Index of Biblical References

Hebrew Bible

Author and Subject Index